# The Aardvark's *Wife*

*An intimate view into the life and challenges of an Asperger marriage*

# The Aardvark's *Wife*

*An intimate view into the life and challenges of an Asperger marriage*

By Carolynn Woods

THE AARDVARK'S WIFE

Copyright © 2009 by Carolynn Woods

All rights reserved

No part of this book may be reproduced in any form or by an electronic or mechanical means, including information storage and retrieval systems, without the permission in writing of the author, except by reviewers in the course of reviewing the book or by print and electronic journalists in the course of reportage on the book and its contents.

Published by Woods Media
Apex, NC

Printed and bound in the United States of America

First Edition

ISBN 978-1448667727

Library of Congress Cataloging-in-Publication Data

Woods, Carolynn.

The Aardvark's Wife/Carolynn Woods

p. cm.

*This book is dedicated to my children,
who will always remain
the brightest part of me.*

# INTRODUCTION

Writing this book took four years to put on paper and twenty-five to construct. In order to chronicle this memoir, I had to revisit the many difficult and painful events which are at the heart of my story. It required periods of recovery from the stressful efforts of retrieving these past experiences and memories in order to authentically describe them. A return visit to an unhappy past is the least anticipated and inarguably the least coveted item on any bucket list.

If you join me in this memoir I must warn it is first, a cautionary tale, and second, it will appear at times to be contradictory and somewhat confusing, but this is the extraordinary nature of the disorder I married.

I wished to accurately illustrate this disorder's uneven and winding path with its abundance of misleading signs and explain why I chose to travel it. Ignorant of the pitfalls and lacking an updated navigational map (which I sincerely hope my story will provide), I was dreadfully unprepared for this solitary expedition into the unknown. This treacherous path I embarked upon was worn from the women who came before and would equally confound those who will follow. We all became lost on this unconventional route of mazes with sharp twists, dizzying turns and no discernable exits; many attempted to carve out a new path only to discover a dead end.

I am not a trained professional in the fields of psychology or developmental disorders. In this personal narrative I present my observations, experiences, thoughts and conclusions for no other purpose than to relate these incredible events to the wives of AS and endow them with the knowledge that they are not alone. I dedicate my story to those who have experienced the same arduous journey. We were unescorted and unrecognized by most. This is a testimony to their struggle and mine with an unidentified and elusive adversary, which proved to be threatening and harmful to our physical and mental health.

I lived with Asperger's Syndrome for twenty-five years; for twenty years it was an unidentified and relentless specter in my life. I wanted to free myself from AS which operated through its host, my husband. It brought me to the brink of mental and emotional collapse. We now live apart, and I am again able to breathe, sleep, and enjoy life as it should be for the first time in a quarter of a century.

Most people are unaware of why this disorder is the suspected cause behind the increase of autism and I will explain why.

I wrote this book for the purpose of revealing the truths, trials, and heartbreak in the life of a woman married to an aardvark.

AARDVARK: Aardvarks are solitary, shy nocturnal animals. Aardvarks live about ten years in captivity; their life span in the wild is unknown. They live in burrows created principally by the female. When aardvarks sleep, they block the entrance to their burrow. If pursued, an aardvark will furiously dig itself a hole. As it is nocturnal and has poor eyesight, the aardvark is cautious upon leaving its burrow, but finally moves out at a slow trot to look for food. Adult aardvarks are solitary, coming together only for mating.

Very little is known about the aardvark and even less about his wife . . .

# CHAPTER 1

*"The people people have for friends your common senses appall, but the people people marry are the queerest folks of all."*

—Charlotte Perkins Gilman

There we stood, just the two of us, in what had become an all too familiar scene. Clay had assumed his "I'm going to have a fit" stance. With his nostrils rapidly flaring and collapsing and his whole body rigid, he vibrated with undiffused anger. His face contorted into the visage of a demon Kabuki mask: eyes bulging and teeth bared for ripping flesh from bone. He stood three feet in front of me, all six-foot-two inches, two hundred-ninety pounds of him. His upper arms clamped to his torso and his forearms extended at waist level in front of him with palms down and his fingers spread wide apart—as if he might manually stop the earth's rotation. I stopped breathing and my heart started pounding. In the span of a second, my body braced for the tangible, yet improbable, threat of a silverback gorilla charge. Normally, I would have run in the face of such a menace, but Clay's rages always caught me by surprise and short-circuited my brain. I froze on the spot where, afterward, I imagined the EMTs would discover my mangled body. Then as suddenly as it was upon me, it was over—a cyclone that had spun itself into oblivion. I was shaken, but alive. The very first time this occurred was about six months after we were married—I had not seen this side of Clay when we were dating and never suspected that this dormant rage even existed.

I had invited three women friends over on a Sunday afternoon to play cards. We were sitting at the table laughing about a misplayed trick. Clay walked in and everyone turned, smiled, and said hello to him. He responded with an icy glare. They shrugged and began quietly talking when suddenly Clay morphed into the l'enfant terrible. We couldn't believe our eyes!

Speechless and terrified by this unprovoked storm from a grown man, they turned their heads from the train wreck unfolding in front of them and looked at me as if to say, why aren't you stopping this? I was in as much of a state of shock as they were. I was dumbfounded. What did he think he was doing? Was this a sick joke?

When all the atoms in the room cooled, he was finally able to articulate his rage in snorted one-syllable words: he couldn't locate a book he had been reading. I was incredulous; I was accustomed to adults asking for help, not tilting the earth on its axis before seeking assistance. I never became immune to the episodes that lasted no more than a few minutes, but learned to expect them. He could, in the blink of an eye, abruptly return to his usual subdued self. I found it hard to accept this as "typical" male behavior. Beneath the reek of testosterone wafted the subtle hint of baby powder—a childish tantrum. He never apologized and those poor traumatized women never came back.

\* \* \*

I recall with great clarity the first time I met Clay. It was New Year's Eve 1982. I was at a singles' party and he was easy to spot—he was taller than the throngs of people huddled together in small friendly groups throughout the clubhouse. Several of my women friends made remarks about the "new guy" and wondered who would be lucky enough to capture his attention.

I was too exhausted from the holidays to play guessing games; I just wanted to go home and curl up with a good book. I had only decided to stay until the bitter end because my girlfriends would have regarded my desire for an early departure as an unforgivable, first-degree transgression. We rode together and they wanted to stay until the dismal, inevitable finale when everyone would shout, "Happy New Year!"

We were a tight group of five divorced mothers who supported and celebrated each other. On the drive home, we became unusually quiet; each one silenced by her own thoughts and regrets on this clear, cold night of disappointment. We warmly hugged each departing friend good night at her home and wished her lots of happiness in the coming year and the man of her dreams. With frail remnants of holiday cheer, we ended another year together.

I didn't see Clay again until we were partnered at our singles' bridge game. I was introduced to him for the first time and couldn't help but notice how everyone there seemed to like this shy, intelligent man.

Several weeks later at a social mixer, we had our first opportunity to talk to each other. While listening to him I thought, how refreshing to find a man who didn't use the standard come-on lines. He was attractive, well groomed and approachable. After a few years of casually dating men who held no matrimonial interest for me, Clay held considerable potential. Later that night he asked me to go out with him. I cannot recall exactly what I said, but I declined.

After eight years as a divorced mother of three, I was reluctant to begin a new relationship, which may or may not go anywhere. I was hesitant to travel down the bumpy road of emotional expenditure and end up alone—again. I felt conflicted with a clot of mixed emotions about dating: finding the time to invest in getting to know someone and the let down when the relationship went south, not to mention the disappointment if I ended up with a real loser.

Then there was always the human need, which ran contrary to the more practical arguments about avoiding emotional suicide: to have that special someone in my life. It was a roller coaster ride and I was certain that I was not up for it, again. Besides, I had reached an enviable level of contentment just being with my children. I found pleasure in the little things; I liked making my own decisions and plans. I liked the freedom of my marketing job with limited travel. I liked my friends and I liked me.

A couple of weeks later, a mutual friend gave Clay my phone number and he called—it took several calls before I relented and accepted one of his invitations to dinner. He cooked for us, nothing elaborate, but I found it endearing that he would attempt to impress me with his limited culinary skill.

I accepted his invitation out of pure desperation: I was bored with staying at home most weekends. It sounds horrible to confess, but on further evaluation of my dating options, I had to accept the fact that a divorced, forty year old woman with three children is usually confined to the shallow end of the dating pool and rarely, if ever, gets the opportunity to dive bikini-clad into the deep end populated with eligible and viable males.

Clay was considerate and attentive. He would call me at work several times a day and although he didn't have much to say, it was flattering to have someone call to just say hello. I sensed from the long pauses on his end telephone conversations weren't his forte. Over the next several months, we spent one or two evenings a week together discussing our shared interests: books, music, movies and occasionally, politics. I came to realize how smart and well-read he was—a fortress of erudition.

He was clearly attracted to me, but never made any sexual overtures, physically or verbally. At first, I was relieved not to have that kind of pressure put on me, but I never considered how this would foreshadow my future relationship with him.

He always made certain we had a date on the weekend. In fact, at times, he was relentless in his pursuit but his efforts seemed genuine and were quite appealing to a single mom. I felt privileged that he was spending so much time with me. The possibility that he was ignoring his friends didn't occur to me since he never mentioned anyone other than his parents or his daughter.

I do remember initiating our first kiss; I had waited for over a month, so I stepped up. I couldn't believe a grown man was that shy, but Clay certainly was. In retrospect I should have considered it strange that a divorced, thirty-eight year old man didn't have any moves. Now, I see clearly that Clay always waited for me to take the initiative in everything. He didn't have a commanding presence, but filled the room with a strange and curious quality that I found somewhat confusing and enticing. It kept me off balance; he was unlike any man I had ever met, but at same time a little familiar, like an eager lost puppy looking for a home. That juxtaposed with the impression that he was something of a man's man—he took karate and was a gun aficionado—made him intriguing—a mystery man. Add a little sprinkle of "dork" and that is a good description of what I saw. Later on, I witnessed his mysterious quality slide smack into the realm of weird.

During our courtship, I didn't notice anything blatantly atypical or abrasive in his character and, truthfully, I wasn't looking, probably because Eros had effectively blinded me. Given the amount of evidence I had at the time, on the surface it appeared that Clay embodied most of the desirable qualities I wanted in a mate. I opened the door to my heart and life to a southern gentleman who was well-mannered, educated, employed, and companionable; all these things made him a standout in any crowd, particularly one made up of single women. He was also accepting and non-judgmental—two big pluses when you're slightly roundish at fortyish.

When he proposed five months into the relationship, he didn't say he loved me, he simply asked if I would like to set a date. I should have held out for a declaration of affection, but I was so surprised that it didn't occur to me to ask for more. I felt I was in love with Clay and wanted to marry again, and he seemed to want this even more than I.

Even after the stormy termination of my first marriage, I hadn't lost my desire or appreciation for marriage. I enjoyed making a home for my family and the addition of a husband/father seemed like the answer to the prayer uttered by many women my age: Please God, don't let me rot on the vine.

Any hesitancy I had about Clay and our short engagement was eagerly sedated by my friends singing a chorus of the old saw, "The first time you choose, the second time you settle." It was true to a great degree. When you are young and have plenty of sexual currency, you can demand a broader, more resplendent slate of candidates for marriage. After the age of forty, you have to narrow your expectations, or least this seemed like the case in the southern climes of 1982. Men of my age had discovered the option of non-committed unions with nubile maidens who were living by a different set of standards from those I was taught: why buy the cow when the milk is free.

The new age and the new morality were exerting a vise-like grip on me to get while the gettin' is good. I had chosen realism over idealism—either way, I was unprepared for what would prove to be neither.

Euphoria or perhaps complacency, two of the sneakier rivals of vigilance, must have distracted me from the salient traits of Clay's true personality. The frustrating truth is there really weren't any discernable red flags particularly when the bride-elect is visually impaired and panting, and specifically when the object of her affection is on his very best behavior.

I easily dismissed many of his quirky habits and odd voice pitch with no intonations except for volume. He didn't seem to have a sense of humor; he got some jokes, but not sarcasm. He didn't know how to respond to affectionate kidding and would just stare at me, uncertain what was expected of him.

My natural willingness to accept some of an individual's idiosyncrasies—unless of course they violated the accepted boundaries of society or plain old good sense, led me right smack into the ride of my life.

At first, Clay's companionship felt comfortable and safe. It was not until we were married, a short six months after we met, that I began to notice a significant divergence in our approach to life. I wasn't going to have good ole uncle so-n-so playing house with me in full view of my children. Therefore, we didn't cohabitate before marriage and Clay's true but hidden personality came as mind-numbing surprises wrapped around little exploding devices that would blow up randomly when I least expected it.

I generously attributed some of his unconventional behavior to different life experiences or perhaps an unusual childhood. As it turned out, it was both and then some.

Never in the history of marriage had there been two more mismatched souls under one roof. Although we were both of the same race and nationality, I had unknowingly entered into a "mixed" marriage to be lived out in an alternative universe and culture where logic was the only spoken language.

## CHAPTER 2

*"Where I am, I don't know, I'll never know, in the silence you don't know, you must go on, I can't go on, I'll go on."*
—Samuel Beckett

A few months into the marriage and after the extinguishment of my prenuptial elation, I felt our marriage was missing something vital to my happiness—passion. Newlyweds, at least in the beginning, engage in nuzzling, pillow talk, titillating phone conversations, and intimate looks. In the weeks after our wedding, we weren't sharing any of these little intimate pleasures—which I had eagerly anticipated.

Clay wasn't affectionate—to the dog, yes, but not with me. He would passively sit still and let me hug or kiss him. It was like making out with a mannequin. He wouldn't close his eyes when we kissed, but instead searched the room to see if anyone was present. It was a timid action, like a child doing something he shouldn't. The bedroom also made him uncomfortable. He acted like he didn't know what to do with me—making me feel like an unsavory chore instead of a lover. I tried to make him feel comfortable and desirable but I soon became exhausted with trying to figure out how to entice him into the bedroom. I'm not saying that he was impotent, he wasn't, but it was close to impossible to get him into bed. I also have to confess that Clay never aroused me; I didn't admit this even to myself until recently—somehow I had missed an obvious lack of sexual chemistry.

I actually believe that if I had said to him, "Honey, we're going to pitch a tent in the bedroom, get some popcorn, tell ghost stories and you can bring the dog," there would have been a real spark of anticipation from him.

I ached for the familiar glances across a crowded room that signaled the desire to be alone and naked. Never once in passing by him did he reach out and pull me into his arms or lap. No afternoon delights. Clay didn't possess the look or language of love. No sweet talk. No flirting. He never shared with me what he was thinking or feeling—ever.

I was frustrated to the point of tears. Aren't most men saturated with testosterone and eager to pursue the female and engage in the "throw down?" I had that impression and like most women, I had personal knowledge that it was the only indisputable fact about a man's nature. Saying "no" is just a minor obstacle to most determined males. Before the "act" comes the sweet talk, the flirting and the cajoling—the silver tongued devil rising up on hind legs, whispering, "Hey, Baby, how about it?" If Clay wanted sex, he sure as heck didn't know how to get it, and it appeared he wasn't eager to try.

These are the examples of his strange behavior that had me scratching my head; he wanted to impress me with his masculinity, but would withdraw when it came down to what I assumed was a mutual and natural desire. It wasn't as though we hadn't had sex before we were married, he knew what he was getting, and I thought he was happy with me; hadn't he confirmed this assumption by marrying me? I had to daily address Clay's neglect for the romantic and the storm it was creating within me. I was a person who wanted to sample as many of life's gifts as possible. Clay was a risk-a-phobic and, I was beginning to suspect, a counterfeit husband.

He was a thinker and I was an incurable romantic. I loved dancing, particularly slow dancing. The stars at night thrilled me with their ominous possibilities, and I could think of nothing more delicious than sitting outside under a canopy of these luminous, astral bodies, cuddled with the love of my life and sharing the dreamspeak of the heavens. I craved curling up by a fire with wine and my favorite vocalists accompanied by a sultry saxophone that shamelessly urged on lovers in the night with abandon and desire. I was a sensual person and every flower, cloud, or the smell of puppy's breath created a pulse in my soul and a desire to share with someone the boundless pleasure of committed love.

I foolishly thought Clay was the person who would co-create this atmosphere of romance. Although he didn't show any outward interest, I must have believed that he was being reserved during our courtship, thinking he was saving up all the good stuff for when we were married. Then we would be free to stagger around our bedroom, tearing off each other's clothes and stumbling over furniture in our hot sweaty attempt to put out the carnal fires that consumed us with such torment. Wrong! That guy never showed up.

I truly believed I was sending standard, "let's make love" signals. Around nine in the evening I would softly whisper in his ear that I was ready for bed; I had to discreetly practice seduction within the confines of a home shared with my three children. He would glance up at me and say, "Okay, good night."

Occasionally, I would try to take advantage of a moment, free from parenting, when we were alone in the house. All of these subtle hints were lost on Clay—the poor guy didn't have a clue when it came to seduction. His total lack of interest and initiative in the bedroom was confusing and hurtful.

My feminine assets were of no interest to him. I hated feeling the shame and rejection of a thwarted lover. It didn't take long for me to discover that sexy lingerie was not only a waste of money, but presentation. My ex-husband had never waited for a signal or an invitation—he was always ready and willing—usually to the extreme. All I had to do was show up and sometimes even that was overkill. I had unknowingly tripped over one of the many indicators of Clay's disorder—this one prevented him from recognizing any signals for intimacy and I wanted to pound him with both fists.

Once when I was feeling dejected and unattractive, I asked, "Honey, do I look fat?" His response was, "Yes." That's all, just "yes." What kind of clod would answer his new bride's need for reassurance with a painfully unmitigated truth? If he felt compelled to tell the truth, a loving response should have been, "Maybe a little, but I still think you're sexy." I never again risked asking for his assessment of me. His cruel remark landed on me like a bag of hammers. I was never safely out of range from his damnable insensitivity. He wasn't intentionally mean; it would without warning burst forth without thought to the damaging consequences that were beginning to undermine our tenuous relationship. I thought it ironic that he was almost one hundred pounds overweight and I was only twenty, but I would have never hurt his feelings by pointing this out.

This change in Clay happened overnight, specifically our wedding night, and it was an abrupt and complete 180 degrees. Where was all the attention and togetherness? Through some cruel agent of alchemy, I had been changed from beloved to insignificant. Later, I thought maybe I was just too sensitive and was imagining these injurious assaults.

The habit of giving him the benefit of the doubt was born right then and there. I tried to shrug off his callous remarks and curb my ebbing self-confidence, which was rapidly becoming a frequent and nearly impossible task since I wasn't receiving any validation by way of compliments or physical reassurances from my new husband. As I look back, I have to acknowledge my ignorance of the obvious: I was living under the assumption that we were two people in love who were living together in a fairly conventional relationship. Mistaken assumption number three and counting...

Because education and intelligence were two of the values imbued in me as a child, and Clay was extremely bright, I had unconscientiously ceded the power of validation over to him.

Genius is a laudable quality; however, love and intelligence share seductive qualities that can lead to blind compliance. I became a candidate for emotional subjugation.

I had been single for a long time and I had spent the last two years of my previous marriage in hell. I came out of that marriage deflated equally in ego and spirit from the cruel rejection incurred by my ex's infidelity and betrayal. Self-induced pressure to recast my past marital failure and to fulfill my present desire to succeed was compelling me to preserve this marriage, which I honestly believed was my last chance for love and happiness.

During a short interval of time, I had witnessed his sudden unprovoked outbursts of anger and puerile frustration, never allayed by an apology, explanation or affectionate reconciliation and his neglect in all the areas of intimacy. Clay remained tuned out and remote. We weren't on the same wave-length and I didn't know why, and if he knew, he wasn't telling me. As smart as he was, I thought, surely he realized something was wrong, and it seemed sadistic to allow someone you supposedly love to turn inside out attempting to please you without giving validation or the merest recognition of their effort.

Clay appeared to stand poised on the precipice of anger—a stick of dynamite with the fuse exposed, waiting for me to strike a match. I never knew what common everyday occurrence would ignite him. He was in his own world, out of reach with his own secret negative stimuli, which I could never decipher. These episodes, like an earthquake, unnerved me. The ground shook under my feet; it then shifted and settled on an unfamiliar vista. Was he Dr. Jekyll or Mr. Hyde? What exactly had I missed in assessing Clay for marriage? In hindsight, I had missed everything! In fairness to me, I was engaged in battle with a hidden disorder. I feel some vindication for my ignorance, but it's small compensation for the years of unhappiness I had to endure before I uncovered what would be a highly elusive truth.

My issues relating to Clay's lack of intimacy and social shortcomings were piling up faster than uncollected garbage. One moment he was kind and solicitous, even docile. The next would be anyone's guess: stony silence, withdrawal, or unprovoked anger. He was not only a stranger, but he was getting stranger every day. In a short three months my new world was shattered; it lay at my feet in disarray, a million scattered pieces begging for an expert hand to reassemble it into a comprehensible mosaic. The marriage seemed to have died before I even had a chance to embrace it. It was traumatic and as painful as the death of a newborn whose arrival was highly and joyously anticipated and then cruelly snatched away.

My first distressing moment came on our wedding night. Clay stayed in the bathroom for over an hour and a half, leaving me alone and wondering, what's taking him so long to come to bed? I finally fell asleep confused and frustrated. The next morning he offered no excuse or an apology for his absence. We quickly consummated our union the next morning—he was in a hurry to eat breakfast!

Job obligations had prevented us from taking a honeymoon. Two days after we married, we were back at work, and on the weekends we were hunting for a house large enough to accommodate a blended family.

Three long months passed before we had sex again. I would slip out of bed in the middle of the night and shower to cover the sobs of despair I feared would awaken the children. I was consumed with panic, confusion and frustration. I began looking at him with a cold and suspicious heart.

Obviously, we were not a typical honeymoon couple: a disinterested groom and a bride who used the bathroom for crying instead of primping. We had both been married before and I knew from my first marriage and from societal norms that most husbands like to exercise their conjugal privileges regularly. Not Clay! Overt sexual rejection and my ever-growing disillusionment with Clay did not bode well for this marriage.

In my effort to try to understand and repair a sinking relationship, a strained and one-sided style of communication began to emerge.

"Clay, what's wrong?"

"Nothing."

"You don't seem to want to make love to me, why?"

"I don't know."

"Did I do something wrong?"

"No."

"Is there someone else?"

"No."

What a question to have to ask a few months after your wedding.

I had many hand-wringing moments when I was willing him to answer, asking him to move into the arena of self-disclosure—he resisted. I had situated us on an emotional plateau; the more I advanced with questions about his feelings, the more he retreated. I envisioned that one day he would eventually back up until he fell off the cliff and I would hang over the edge shouting to him, "Why couldn't you just answer the stupid question?" The only conversations Clay was mildly willing to engage in were those that centered on non-personal issues. Our dialogue sounded strained—short, impersonal and solely informational as though we had been married for decades instead of weeks.

He introduced me to strangers as "My wife," with the same vocal intonation as, "This is my car" or "My watch." Clay sounded like someone had filtered out all the emotion from his voice.

Left with so many unanswered pleas for insight, I surmised it had to be something about me and he was hesitant to mention it. There had to be something I was guilty of doing or perhaps not doing. I assumed I was the only other person in the equation. Was I undesirable, too fat, too short, too dumb? Evidently, since I was a woman it was my duty to take the blame for the relationship's failure—the cultural conditioning of my generation, which had taught us to be responsible for men's behavior, had not been lost on me. He offered no explanations about what was bothering him and impeding our love life, and he appeared unconcerned about addressing or repairing it.

Clay was like a new book with a rigid spine—it could not be forced open for perusing; it would just spring shut and remain an enigma. I learned that no answer is the cruelest answer.

I felt deeply discouraged after only a few months into the marriage; the intimacy and communication had stopped—more accurately, it hadn't begun. When one partner is playing twenty questions with no participation by the other, everything is up for speculation. In the absence of his input, I thoroughly and painfully dissected myself and saw no conceivable reason why I should receive this unkind, insensitive treatment.

Forced to draw my own conclusions, I determined he was gay. That would explain his effete mannerisms and the avoidance of intimacy in the bedroom. It was the only thing in this marital charade that made sense. That was my initial conviction and although later proven inaccurate, it satisfied my immediate quandary over Clay's sexual orientation and lack of libido.

This was the first in a long line of sustainable, but agonizing rationalizations; each interlocking with the preceding one until they created an ironclad chain, which eventually anchored me in a marriage to a man who was beyond comprehension within any known context.

CAROLYNN WOODS

## CHAPTER 3

*"Curiouser and curiouser!"*

—Lewis Carroll

Clay had a daughter and I had three children from our previous marriages. Blending these two distinctly different families would prove to be a monumental and stressful undertaking. Maintaining my emotional equilibrium would prove to be an even greater task.

Melinda, Clay's ten-year-old daughter, was sweet, but spoiled (but then many "only" children are). She threw tantrums when she didn't get what she wanted and preferred to play alone. Perhaps preferred was not a correct assumption; it seemed, sadly, that she was doomed to play alone. She didn't have any friends. My children, two teenage daughters and a ten-year-old son, liked Clay—the definitive test for any of my past beaus—and in the same spirit, they tried to embrace Melinda. She would test our ability to establish a blended family, where everyone would feel loved, accepted and valued. I had no experience with children like Melinda. She defied every parenting method I knew.

Whenever people live under the same roof there must be some consensus on how to meet the daily demands of lifestyle, parenting, setting boundaries, fiscal responsibility, the fulfillment of individual needs and equally important—emotional support. Between Clay's enigmatic lifestyle and Melinda's behavioral problems, I had to throw all the standard conventions for structuring a "normal" life out the window and begin with very elementary steps.

Attempting to parent someone else's child is a perilous and unrewarding venture in the best of circumstances, but this was to be a constant and abusive test of my patience and strength. A stepparent is in a "no win" situation no matter how sincere and loving the intention. Melinda's odd nature continues to escape me to this day.

Before we were married, I had suggested to Clay perhaps family counseling would be helpful since we had four children to assimilate into one family. He declined without an explanation.

Clay had settled into what I assumed was his parenting style from his previous marriage—let someone else do it. He would pontificate about how he and his ex had parented (I suspected it was mainly his ex), and he expected me to continue in the same liberally indulgent tradition. Clay appeared to have a genuine concern for the children, but was clueless and ineffective as a parent. Often, because of his childish behavior, I tossed him in the soup with the kids. The only way to tell them apart—he was the one with the beard and car keys. Whenever the children got into a row, Clay would jump in and have a "finger-spreading" fit. I told him to stop interfering. Someone (me) needed to resolve these conflicts between siblings in an adult fashion, all Clay did was redirect attention to himself by jumping into the fray clueless as to what caused the argument or how to resolve it. It looked as if he didn't know what else to do, but needed to be a part of the negative energy. Naturally, when there is a nearly three hundred pound man wildly flapping around the room it's easy to lose the initial focus. After dealing with Clay's fit and sending him off to pout somewhere, I would be right back to the original feuding issue between siblings, only now I was exhausted and wanted to shoot them all.

Melinda and Clay were two speed bumps in our lives; whenever we planned to do anything as a family, like a vacation or eat out, we would have to slow down and overcome their hesitancy to change focus or location. Clay was only concerned with expense and Melinda never wanted to do anything as a group—it was their lack of spontaneity I resented the most. Clay and Melinda weren't in the least embarrassed to have one of their feuds in public. I was horrified the first time it happened. Naturally, it was about Melinda not getting something she wanted, and she would throw a fit in front of God and everybody, screaming at her father in hopes he would give in. They would volley back and forth, back and forth, with the same diatribe. He had also dug in and was not about to allow Melinda into his wallet. I would sneak away to some spot where I could watch them, but not be readily associated with the Hatfields and McCoys. They were victim to the only two vocal emotions either of them could express—anger and frustration. They appeared to lack the internal social filters which should have prevented them from displaying this behavior in public. They had to have center stage and the big spotlight. Their conduct stated that they were the only two people in the universe and their needs should be the immediate and total focus of the planet. I was pulled in so many directions at once—please the husband, keep his ex off my back by placating the demanding, spoiled stepdaughter, and at the same time consider my children and their needs. I could feel the tightening grasp of stress slither around my body like a giant boa constrictor squeezing the life out of me. It was too much for anyone to handle in a family with only one adult parent and five children, plus or minus the bearded one.

It was particularly difficult to convince Melinda to share anything, whether it was TV time, toys or treats. She had to have her own things, which in an ideal world is great, but as a family, we couldn't afford for everyone to have their own TV. She was like Clay; if someone wanted to borrow or share something of theirs, they would recoil, sharing was unacceptable. Clay and Melinda particularly resented sharing food. They were self-contained units; there would be no mingling of possessions. Clay, the tightwad, would even offer to go out and buy the item in dispute when we couldn't afford it rather than feel forced to share it.

Melinda was ten years old when we married and couldn't make her own sandwich or pour a bowl of cereal. She still carried her "blankie" with her when she came to stay with us. I didn't make an issue of it as I felt she might need this security object until she felt more at home with us.

My children had demonstrated independence much younger. They were making their own sandwiches at the age of five or six—not neatly or nutritiously, but the effort was there and they were so proud of themselves for being self-reliant.

In our second summer together, we planned to go to the beach for a week's vacation—a well deserved break for everybody. Melinda was coming with us and I was happily expecting family bonding to take place on neutral territory. My girls were excited and I could tell my son harbored secret expectations of mentoring by a "real" dad who would teach him to surf, fish, or just hang out and do "guy" stuff. As soon as we settled into the beach house, Clay plopped down in a chair and began to read. The only interruptions he tolerated were mealtimes and my requests to placate Melinda when she was having a tantrum. Evidently, we all had personal and conflicting expectations about what a real family would do on vacation.

Naturally, Melinda saw her father as her own personal property, present exclusively to cater to her demands. This was to be expected, but Clay didn't view the situation as an opportunity to bring us all closer together and simply functioned as Melinda's keeper and an outsider to us. I kept house, cooked and herded the brood covered in sand and sunscreen to the beach and back. At the end of the day, I envisioned taking a long walk on the beach in the moonlight with Clay; I took a long walk alright—alone. Although we were under the same roof, it was separate vacations for us as a couple.

When I packed for our trip, I brought food and games and gave each one of the young'uns their own giant box of cookies, to avoid squabbling over the goodies. Proud of my cleverness to avert a melee over sharing, I was stunned to discover that Melinda would rise early every morning and spend twenty minutes, first lining up and then counting and recounting her cookies. I'm not certain what the particular consequence would have been if she had come up short, but I am certain it would have been a dilly. Clay and Melinda reminded me of a dog we once had who guarded food; if we came within two feet of his food dish, he let out a low guttural growl and bared his teeth. It wasn't as though we couldn't go to the store to buy more, but she had a deep sense of ownership for those cookies. Melinda and her father placed more value on things than people. She accumulated toys, mostly stuffed animals, and hoarded them, but she seemed to find little pleasure in these possessions. My children had enjoyed their toys and games most when playing with others; they had a hard time understanding Melinda's reluctance to play or share with them.

This child was smart, but I felt that maybe she was also a little retarded and a little feral. She would sit in front of the television for hours with her mouth hanging open and a blank expression on her face—disconnected and alone.

Melinda didn't strike me as a happy child. She never did anything with wild abandon or pure joy, but then neither did her father—they were serious people. She was bossy and a tattletale and so was her father. She would come running to me with petty complaints. Any confrontations had to be resolved in a manner that appeased Melinda. Out of sheer exasperation, I finally told her to settle her own problems, and she did—with screams, tantrums or physical violence. She had no negotiating skills. She solved conflicts with my son by scratching him until he bled. Neither she nor her father could repair an altercation, nor did they give the impression that it was very high on their list to learn how. It was very difficult for me to watch as she tortured my children with her selfish, violent actions. I could not punish her. Melinda wasn't held accountable for her actions by her parents, and I wasn't going to step into that trap. She would give me a hug when prompted to do so, and she appeared to want to engage my children, but expected them to fill the role of doting, tolerant parents, always giving in to her demands. I really didn't know how to relate to her, and I couldn't tell anyone about my problems with her. I thought people would believe I was overly sensitive to her spoiled behavior or resented her for being part of Clay's past, but the truth was I did feel affection for her; I just didn't know how to live with her. If I had not been so distracted most of time, I would have known Melinda was a child with special needs. I thought it was strange when Clay with his military background couldn't handle the disciplinary problems presented by a ten year old. Later, much later, I learned why they were so similar in behavior.

I was grateful for one small insight from Clay regarding Melinda. He told me when Melinda was a young child in daycare, she was taught to tell an adult when she had a problem with another child—which was usually precipitated by her biting and scratching. Maybe it was appropriate instruction when she was three or four, but she was nearly eleven and needed to learn some self control and social skills. On many days, I spent my energy avoiding the two of them. I quickly became disillusioned with the whole "blended family" concept. These two "aliens" on our family planet were beyond assimilating. They had reduced me to a whimpering lump, and I had two hormonal, teenage daughters, who were cuddly puppies compared to Clay and Melinda. At least my daughters' adolescent behavior was predictable. I could manage the upheaval these two teenagers created; I knew there were parenting resources, if I needed them—and I did. It was in the uncharted waters concerning Clay and Melinda that I was having the most difficulty. I had no navigational charts tacked on the wall for quick references or fixes. Never at any time did I feel their behavior was intentional or directed toward making my life a living hell, nor did I feel any evil plot to destroy the family was "afoot," evidently this was their bizarre nature.

To exacerbate the situation, Clay's ex would call to tell him how I should punish my son when he responded to Melinda's violent behavior. He called her a "bitch" the first time she drew blood. My son never used this language, but I could understand his frustration, and he was punished—but by my rules. Melinda, as always, escaped punishment or reprimand. As uncomfortable as her behavior was to my family, her parents and grandparents tolerated it.

I was able to convince Clay to tell his ex we would handle our family (exaggerated optimism on my part) and she should handle hers. Clay always managed to remain aloof, while the rest of us flawed mortals wailed at the wall in an effort to make sense of these two, very strange aliens in our lives.

I was now the linchpin of the family—that in itself was scary, since I was on the brink of falling apart. My days would end not in the safe haven of a husband's loving and consoling arms, but in the bleak isolation of a cold bed.

## CHAPTER 4

*"The place where optimism most flourishes is in the lunatic asylum."*
—Havelock Ellis

I loved Clay and Melinda and wanted to make them a welcomed part of my family and I expected the same from them. But, sadly, they didn't know how or perhaps saw no personal benefit in reciprocating this gesture—it felt like the latter. They both had a strong sense of entitlement—they could act without consideration and were oblivious to the actions we saw as inappropriate. I willingly opened up my family, inserted Clay and Melinda, and stitched up the kindred fabric as seamlessly as possible, but there was always a loose thread—one small tug and I feared it was going to rip apart.

Shortly after my son turned eleven, a faculty member at his school overheard him confiding to a friend that he wanted to commit suicide. This was a serious wake-up call. By that afternoon, we were sitting in the office of a child psychiatrist. Obviously, we would both need counseling. I was deeply concerned about my son and was impatient to hear the doctor's evaluation, and I was scared. Suppose no one overheard him. I was trying to follow the doctor's assessment while reminding myself to breathe. I had to be present on every level to comprehend what she was about to tell me. I felt guilty, too. During my mangled efforts to balance a new life with two new personalities and problems, I managed to almost lose my son. He was lost in the turmoil created when I was trying to juggle a life with new husband and a part time stepdaughter, and the nightmares inherent with trying to cover all the bases with only one outfielder.

My son, Mark, was having difficulty adjusting to our new family's lifestyle, but with counseling sessions for us both, we would be fine, his counselor stated. Did she say fine? I didn't feel fine and thought I would probably never feel fine again. At least for the present, my son was out of harm's way and we would continue counseling for at least a year. I still thank God every day for our recovery from a potential tragedy.

Mark had no relationship with his father and put high hopes on Clay filling those shoes, but like me, soon realized that this was a futile wish. Clay wasn't a father to his own daughter. He seemed to care about the children, but was clueless and ineffectual as a parent. My son took this rejection from his own father and more recently from Clay as an indication of his self-worth. Of course, I was doing the very same thing. I, too, had expected Clay to function in a parental role as well as a spouse. I thought as an adult, I had more mature and sophisticated tools for working through this than a child of eleven did. I didn't.

For many months we faithfully continued with counseling, I with my counselor and my son with his. A progress report on my son's sessions followed each appointment. I felt encouraged; he seemed like a different child, happy and hopeful. He liked sports and became involved with more activities outside the home with my support and supervision.

My counselor and I were trying to explore the problems in the marriage; I didn't have to dig too deeply. My counselor, an older woman, wanted to explore my relationship with Clay, to determine what was causing me so much confusion and stress. I told her about our problems and my suspicions. It was the first time I had repeated my litany of complaints to a professional; even to me it sounded petty, not to mention paranoid, but I bravely soldiered on trying to remember every insult or injury Clay had perpetrated on my psyche. It was not easy for me to air my dirty laundry, especially about my marriage, to anyone. I felt I had failed—to be a good mother and wife. Failure was beginning to feel like a fashion accessory—accenting and defining me.

When I told her about Clay's neglect of our sex life, or rather the lack of one, the good doctor looked at me as if I had casually mentioned that I had a fly in my soup. She matter-of-factly informed me that men who did not want to have sex with women were either gay or pedophiles. What? My brain sputtered. Didn't this deserve a little more investigation—maybe an interview with Clay? I sat silent, in utter disbelief. I was shaken inside and out. Yes, I had thought he might be gay, but coming from a professional it sounded conclusive—no room left for speculation. The guessing game was over; I had married either a homosexual or a pedophile.

Although I still had many other unanswered questions about Clay, it wasn't about me anymore; it was about my children's safety. I had a son who may be in danger of molestation by someone I brought into our lives! His counselor assured me that there was no evidence of sexual violation—by anyone. I took a deep breath and gave a prayer of thanks, but my relief deserted me when I realized I still had two teenage daughters who might be the actual targets of perversion. I had had talks with my children about sexual predators, and I was pretty confidant the girls, who were older than their brother, were perceptive and would report any improprieties to me. I wasn't so naïve that I didn't know about these scenarios—a stepfather who took liberties with available young girls. I knew Clay had a stash of pornography so I sped home and tore through the offensive pile of "literature," looking for anything that would indicate if he had a penchant for little boys or underage girls.

Queasy and repulsed by the nature of his reading material, I was relieved that he had nothing which hinted at pedophilia.

I grew suspicious too as to why, whenever Melinda came for a visit, her grandmother and mother hovered via the phone to check on her well-being; I assumed it was to see if I, the "evil" stepmother, had shaved her head or set her on fire. I even entertained the thought that they may have suspected Clay harbored a dark side when it came to his daughter, but in a less panicky moment, thought perhaps they lacked confidence in Clay's parenting abilities. I felt confident it was the latter. After all, who knew him better than his ex-wife or his mother?

That evening when we were alone, I confronted Clay about his sexual orientation. He assured me he was heterosexual and was only interested in women of legal age. What women? Did he mean, any woman, but me? He sounded sincere when he told me he was heterosexual and I believed him. I wanted to believe him. However, I did threaten him with legal repercussions and physical harm if he ever transgressed the parent-child bond. He was shocked, but, surprisingly, not angry I would consider him capable of such depravity.

Aside from this momentary vindication from sexual misconduct, I didn't dare retract my maternal antennae. I would have to remain vigilant every minute of every day. The trust was fading into gross suspicions and I hated it; it added to the burgeoning load of stress already homesteading on my shoulders.

In the absence of openness and communication, I was running amok with speculations about who Clay was and what he was capable of doing. I felt terrible. I really needed to share with someone who had been through a similar ordeal, had I even known of anyone, but I was still hesitant to discuss my bungled life with anyone. I felt ashamed and very confused.

I quit my job; monitoring the lives of my children became my immediate priority and the daily bouts of diarrhea weren't helping. Not coincidently, my health was beginning to react to these many new assaults from fear and doubt. Irritable bowel syndrome, migraines and hypertension, new and unwelcome additions to my life alternately plagued me, making it impossible for me to work. I didn't know what to do or where to go for help, normally I would have turned to my husband, but he was the problem.

Clay countered my hysteria with rational arguments; he was good at mitigating any circumstance so it didn't disturb his status quo, and he could convince me it was the right thing to do. Financially, it was impossible for us to divorce—it always seemed to come down to money; we had no way of knowing when we would sell the house, and we could not survive on his income alone. His arguments made sense but didn't change the nagging feeling of being handed a prison sentence.

This was a never-ending quagmire of circumstances: a marriage less than two years old that was definitely in a downward spiral, a financial fiasco, my health, and the impact on the children, whom I felt needed constant protection. I began having Freudian-style night terrors. I dreamed I was trying to run from an unseen villain, but my body felt heavy and unresponsive. I woke up in a cold sweat with screams constricted in my throat, certain that I had awakened the whole household, but I heard only my muffled whimpers coming from deep within.

Next to me, Clay slept serenely undisturbed. I directed my anger toward him for two reasons: he was not sharing this hellish existence, and when I tried to talk to him about it, he was detached and unaffected by the human drama and the resulting trauma I was experiencing. He showed no concern, offered no compassion or even entertained a mild curiosity about what was making me so unhappy and causing me so much stress. I came to believe I was invisible to him.

CAROLYNN WOODS

# CHAPTER 5

*"Genius is an infinite capacity for giving pains."*
—Don Herold

It was 1984 and nothing had changed for the better in my life with Clay, however, across the Atlantic in the U.K., Dr. Lorna Wing, a British psychiatrist, was writing a book based on the work of a Viennese pediatrician using his observations of the children he treated in his clinic during the Second World War. This scholarly work would become my Rosetta Stone.

Unfortunately, it would be another ten years before her work would make its way to the medical community in the U.S. and establish a new and devastating diagnosis. Getting the long awaited answers about Clay's odd behavior would remain years out of my reach. In the interim, I continued to struggle with the chaos his disorder created.

I went back to work. I started a small business and used this venture as a cloak I could wrap myself in to avoid spending too much time with Clay.

On the surface, Clay appeared to understand the daily operation of a household, but his eccentric habits were not easy to ignore or integrate into the flow of a typical lifestyle. He would deliver suggestions pleasantly and I, suffering from terminal "please" disease, would comply. He thought alphabetizing all the canned goods and spices in the kitchen cabinets would be a splendid idea—it seemed like a logical and benign request, except he expected me to do it. He also wanted the dishes placed in the dishwasher in a prescribed manner. He ran into resistance with this chore since it was my children's, their preferred method required speed, not organization. Every evening after dinner, highly agitated Clay would rearrange the dishes according to his system while we watched. The nightly hassle became too much for us to endure so we fled to the opposite end of the house. Distance was a good salve.

My grandfather was blind for most of his adult life and my grandmother structured everything in their lives around his disability. She arranged the furniture to facilitate his movements throughout the house. She spent hours rearranging the food staples, bath supplies, tools and anything else he might need while she was at work. As streamlined as these conveniences were, he constantly called upon her to find, hand or fetch something for him. She was a prisoner to his demands. We all lived with the same arrangement of furniture and wound our way through life with the constraints dictated by his handicap. Now I was in the same position all over again and I did it willingly, but never stopped to consider—Clay wasn't handicapped, or was he? Obliviously, I was going to make this marriage work even if it killed me and it nearly did.

I was aware of the big changes caused by Clay and Melinda, but was unaware of subtle changes taking place all around me and unless they became big enough to cause me to trip and slam headlong into a wall, I missed them on a conscious level. I was working, taking care of the house and lawn, and raising three or four children depending on which weekend it was, and catering to a husband who was oblivious to the fact that I was doing all the above—without help. My body and mind were sending signals I had no time to interpret. I was absorbing the bombardment of silent, stealthy toxins into my body and mind as effortlessly as an odorless noxious gas.

Everyone in my life was demanding more and more and giving less and less. I couldn't stop long enough to assess the damage this unrealistic lifestyle would cost me. The financial security and benefits Clay brought to the marriage certainly helped maintain a family. By now, I knew it was solely up to me to keep this family together and I knew if I stopped doing any of the many things I did, my children would suffer and this house of cards would collapse.

Clay wanted to go to the grocery store with me, and since I was working and food shopping was a real chore, I welcomed the help. What had been a thirty to forty-five minute errand quickly turned into an hour and a half combat mission—most men would rather spend that amount of time having sex, not Clay, he preferred pushing a shopping cart down grocery aisles. Regardless of where I was in the store, he would call me and I would come running to see what he wanted. He then rummaged through the cart of products I had collected and insisted I divide ounces into cents to determine the best price on each item. I began sneaking off from work early to avoid this "buddy" system of shopping.

Clay took frugality to an Olympic level of competition. He suggested I buy gas at a certain station. It didn't matter that it was ten miles out of the way; he thought we could save two cents a gallon on gas. I have no objections to economizing, and I am certainly not extravagant, but he took it to a new standard that even I couldn't rival. Shopping and suggesting new chores for me appeared to be Clay's newest hobbies; his demands were logical and practical and I couldn't argue with that, but they were oppressive.

There was never room for spontaneity. He never said, "Hey, honey, let's leave this mess and go to the movies!" If he saw the tired, harangued woman scrubbing floors, mowing the lawn, hanging wallpaper, or grooming the dog and who desperately needed something to relieve the ongoing stress in her life, he never acknowledged it or attempted to change it. He never came to me and took the mop out of my hand and led me to a chair and said, "You sit and let me finish."

One weekend I took off work and painted and wallpapered the entire kitchen. A friend of mine came by to admire the decorating job and as she "oohed" and "aahed" over my handiwork, Clay proudly announced we did it. If I could have raised my exhausted arms, which hung limply by my sides, high enough to reach his throat… I remember shooting him a "look," which he either didn't see or didn't understand, probably both. He often took credit for things I had done and showed no shame for doing it.

He would log in the mileage for his car every time he bought gas. "Why?" I asked. He wanted to determine miles per gallon, he replied. "Yes, but after three years with the same car and driving approximately the same distance to and from work, wouldn't it be a constant every week?" "Yes." Even in the face of this flawless logic, he still slavishly entered the numbers in his little black book. It was an inane ritual. I was becoming painfully familiar with inane exercises—mine and his.

Our life had become predictable, uncomfortable and boring. There were always injured feelings to soothe and tempers to defuse, which usually arose from minor misunderstandings. We spoke two different languages. I lean toward non-verbal expressions: eye signals, a nod of the head, a smile or a grimace—believing at some point in a relationship, a shorthand style of communication emerges—wrong again! Clay had only two modes of communication: talking or fit throwing, whichever required the big spotlight.

Clay was a creature of habit; any deviation from his norm could cause a domestic calamity and elicit a weak, rapid heart rate. He couldn't switch back and forth from one activity to another, either by choice or from an interruption. If he was involved in something and I had to interrupt him, I dreaded his response. He confided once that he and his temper had quite a reputation in his workplace. On the other hand, he felt free to intrude upon me whenever he felt the need. When I was watching a television program, he felt entitled to walk into the middle of the room, stand in front of me and demand my attention, without apology, "I can't find my beige socks." "Do you need them right now?" "No, but I want to know where they are." If I was in the bathroom, and the phone rang, he would knock on the door announcing, "It's for you." "Okay, Clay, can you tell them I'll call back?" My children did this to me until they were eight or nine years old and finally the reality of the situation kicked in, and they were able to judge when it was better to take a number and leave me with a shred of dignity. After twenty-five years, Clay continued to bring the phone to the bathroom door.

It was strange and injurious to me how he could ignore my feelings and needs, but nothing escaped his attention when it concerned him. A missing book, a misplaced pen, or my car parked on the wrong side of the garage. These incidents were cause for disrupting our lives to deliver an explanation for the transgression. He was the biggest pain whenever he felt he was losing control over either a situation or his possessions.

We all learned to take a back seat to Clay's unyielding and demanding attitude. I concluded that since Clay had been an officer in the U.S. Army, he was likely constrained by a military mindset. He never saw combat during the Viet Nam war, but served in Turkey as an intelligence officer; perhaps that would explain why he was so uncommunicative and regimented. Clay held a degree in applied mathematics. The fact he had a methodical, albeit, inflexible manner of thinking, made sense considering this background. However, I was still not satisfied that this was the only explanation for Clay's subjective and maddening behavior. I grew up in a military family and we managed to be flexible and spontaneous, we even had fun.

Even though I had been deluded into thinking he was heterosexual, before we were married he asked his mother to make him a red velveteen, floor length caftan which he proudly wore around the house. He also instructed me on the preferred way to make any dish that came out of the kitchen. "It's okay, but maybe next time you could add more of . . ." These weren't suggestions about how to improve something, but directives; compliments were non-existent in the marriage; his whole family was remiss in this flattering gesture.

I would invite him to take evening walks with me in the neighborhood, and he insisted on carrying a tall walking stick to fend off potential attacks by barking, tail wagging dogs who were excited to see neighbors. I had to convince him that a simple "shoo" could accomplish the desired results and eventually the stick stayed at home.

The bedroom was still the only room in the house with a single purpose—sleep. He lay beside me in bed, reading Playboy magazine, and totally ignored the available and willing woman beside him. I would think to myself, who are you, man, woman or child? He was presenting me with confusing split images and it was driving me bonkers. When I couldn't find answers to the question: "who" he was, I was willing to turn the microscope on me. What in heaven's name was I doing to deserve this hurtful neglect?

Our sex life dwindled to a damp, gasping ember. At first, we had sex three or four times a year, then twice a year, then we skipped years. Finally these long intervals turned into abstinence. I asked how he could go for years without wanting to make love, "I guess I'm not as needy as you are," he arrogantly mused. It has been eighteen years since our last sexual encounter. I never considered myself sexually addicted, but compared to him—I was beginning to wonder. He was thirty-eight and I was forty-two, and I wasn't ready to give up my love life. I was angry, hurt, and confused over being forced into a life of sexual abstinence. He refused to discuss this subject and left me out in the cold with the sting of rejection, again. I did not fit into this man's life in any way I could fathom other than that of a dedicated servant. I had been gradually and extrinsically transformed from a woman into an artifact.

## CHAPTER 6

*"A healthy male adult bore consumes each year one and a half times his weight in other people's patience."*
—John Updike

The ultimate revelation about Clay didn't come to me for many years. Its discovery was agonizingly incremental—layer by layer, stone by stone, and splinter by splinter. I felt I was rebuilding the Egyptian pyramids single-handed. This was a costly endeavor in terms of time, energy, and emotional expenditure; it damaged my health and destroyed by self-confidence. This had ceased to be a labor of love, but rather an exercise in survival. I had to narrow my search down to minute bites so as not to choke on huge chunks of disorienting information. First, I needed to determine what I was married to, a man or a child. But before I could resolve that question, a hundred more were queuing up and urgently demanding my immediate attention, I was driven by panic and many unmet needs, I wanted to be loved and accepted by the man I married.

I wanted to ask him questions about his strange behavior, but this time I decided to ask about his past. I stopped asking him about how he felt about me. He was willing to disclose any information that accentuated his intellect or that wasn't of an emotional nature, if we ran into an intimate area, he closed up tighter than a clam. I tried very hard to avoid the intimate, but for me, that was the essence of emotional nurture, and I craved it like oxygen. Over time my questions stacked up and remained in a holding pattern, hovering menacingly over my head. I had to learn what and how to ask.

I thought maybe having friends over would lighten the gloom surrounding my marriage; I invited them over for cookouts, sit-down dinners, or cards—anything that helped me avoid being alone with Clay. Clay's company was the loneliest lonely I had ever endured. He tolerated my friends' visits rather well. But when I asked him about inviting his friends, his answer startled me. He had none. I had missed some very important chapters in his life because he never talked freely about his past or people. I asked him about high school friends and it seems there weren't any. I inquired about his college friends—none! Where were his Army buddies? Again, nope.

Clay had no close or even casual friends—evidently, I was it and I wasn't too happy with him. More than a little alarmed, I moved on to his dating history. Nope, nothing there either. He never had a "real" girlfriend. He hung out at home with his parents and read. He ate, slept, and read. He never had a job after school or during summer breaks. Also missing from his life experiences were hobbies, sports, scouting, camping and dating. He attended college while living at home. He had a short stint in an apartment with two other students, but that didn't last long.

He met his ex-wife, a computer science major, in their junior year and they married after graduation.

I asked him about his interests and activities as an adolescent, he answered, "Reading." As a child he read the same genres as he does as an adult. He read science fiction, fantasy, medieval history, astronomy, and U.S. military history. His whole world only existed on the printed page. His only adolescent sexual encounters were from the pages of Playboy.

Clay had a younger brother, three years his junior, who was his primary playmate. Between childhood and his engagement, the sum total of his social history was a blank page. Once during a fanciful escape from reality, I thought an alien spacecraft delivered Clay to earth and his parents raised him as a hybrid human. I wasn't too far off base.

Clay had attained the rank of Captain in the U.S. Army. After separating from the military, he moved back to his hometown with his wife and settled down to a career in information technology.

He enjoyed my friends and seemed to like having them over—fresh meat for his lectures, but he eventually drove them away with his long-winded discourses, which centered solely on his special interests.

My women friends weren't in the least interested in Star Wars technology or medieval weaponry, but Clay was not above hijacking any conversation we were engaged in and turning it into the direction of his interests. He was not only disinterested and critical of the subjects offered by our guests, but also highly intolerant of any opposition to his theories and opinions. It was his arrogance and imperious attitude, which accompanied these diatribes as much as anything, not to mention the occasional "fit" that sent our poor guests stampeding to the door with vague excuses for an early exit.

The inevitable post mortem that followed these dinner parties gave me an opportunity to explain to a perplexed Clay why everyone left abruptly. I explained to him how most people enjoy exposure to new information, but resent having it shoved down their throats by an insensitive host.

He sat quietly and let me tutor him in the nuances of social skills; I even thought he was taking my comments to heart, but his eyes would dart all around the room. Was it boredom or avoidance? Like a blast of arctic air, the revelation froze me in mid-thought—he couldn't make eye contact. Once more unaware, I had stumbled into the labyrinth of Clay's disorder. It broke my heart to think that the man who had seen me naked couldn't look me in the eye.

He always promised, with the same child-like sincerity, to change, to do better. Of course, it never happened—he was incapable of change.

Clay didn't understand the natural course of social conversation or about the rhythm and a flow that takes place when people exchange information. People use the elements of this highly social practice for the purposes of sharing experiences, information and bonding. Conversation, or at least Clay's interpretation of it, was for the sole purpose of relating volumes of dry factual data without an iota of consideration of how this juggernaut bearing down on them made them feel. He was unintentionally rude and could occasionally be brutal.

When I tried to share some new insight or discovery with him, I was met with the same arrogant response, "I know." Then he would proceed to correct me in the presence of our guests. I gave up talking when he was around. Clay never allows anyone else to have the last word. I found myself forced into the position of only nodding in agreement like a well-trained toady. He treated me with such disregard; I felt like an idiot incapable of intelligent speech or thought. My feelings were secondary to Clay's need to be the center of attention. Petulant and overbearing are the best descriptors of his social demeanor. Finally, I began to understand his lack of friends. He did not know how to play with the other kids; he was too old to be a child and too socially immature to behave as a considerate and sensitive adult.

Clay's contentment came at a dear cost to me; either he was reading and ignoring me or holding me hostage with his need to show off his intellect. His only language style was informational and impersonal, which spewed out of him regardless of his audience. In between engagements he was taking in more data, to be processed (a habit I called "data dosing") and regurgitated back to the unsuspecting. He would subject the people standing in line at the post office or the movies to his opinions and knowledge without benefit of sotto voce. I was mortified as heads turned and stared at us, but it never occurred to him to feel embarrassed. He preferred just the two of us alone where at his leisure he could deliver his nightly reports. My only function was to be a captive audience. His body language reminded me of a child who was unaccustomed to speaking in public. If standing, he shifted his weight from one foot to the other, fidgeting nervously, and the entire time his eyes ricocheted around the room. He would not look directly at me. I kept looking in the direction of his line of vision to see what had grabbed his attention. Before I could determine what it was, he was off again looking at anything but me.

He reported on the weather, national and international news, politics, and science. When he ran out of all the former topics, he began with mundane, household inventories: "We need milk, toilet paper, Kleenex and light bulbs." Now these items couldn't be just run-of-the-mill generic products we had to research them for longevity, price per unit, etc. My response to this nightmare was an overwhelming desire to run through the streets screaming at the top of my lungs, "Kill me—kill me now!"

Everyday the information super highway, all six lanes of it, ran through my living room. His voice, devoid of tonal inflection and emotion, would drone on until I made an excuse to leave the room or go to bed. At times, death seemed like a merciful solution to my angst. My interests, my needs or me, were not subjects under consideration for discussion. It never occurred to Clay that I found no joy in the relationship. He was unaware that the arrangement we shared was not a marriage by any definition other than legal.

I was never a wife or a soul mate. I was a utility. I was a live-in cook, housekeeper, captive audience, and an imprisoned human being without the promise of parole.

CAROLYNN WOODS

## CHAPTER 7

*"One may understand the cosmos, but never the ego; the self is more distant than any star."*
—G.K. Chesterton

As the years dragged and flew by, I continued to wonder why Clay married me. Since he wouldn't offer any reason for this unconventional and sexless union between us, I took it upon myself to find some psychological explanation for this weird man who through his strange actions and lack of interpersonal communication had negated the opportunity for a successful and happy marriage.

One evening, a few months into the marriage, he stood at the back door ready to take out the trash when I realized he was waiting for something; I looked over at him when he asked me to open the door for him, seeing that he held the trash bag with only one hand, I had to ask, "What's wrong with your other hand?" He looked down to discover that indeed he did have a free hand and could open the door for himself. I remembered when I was growing up and heard discussions about people who had "book sense," but no common sense. Recalling this conversation I thought so this is what they look like! Yes, I was married to one, but I couldn't believe God had made only one. Surely, there had to be others.

I began a pathless journey into the world of clinical labels, which I thought might offer some insight into how Clay's mind worked or rather, didn't work. I went through the long list of personality disorders: narcissism (I put a check mark by that one), bi-polar disorder, multiple personalities (checked that one), schizophrenia, arrested development (I put two checks by that one). Some characteristics seemed to apply, but there never was an exact fit. I knew after twelve years that I was dealing with something pathological, but what? I didn't have a clue. On one level, he was a grown man gifted with extreme intellectual capabilities and, simultaneously, as helpless and clueless as a child. He was polite and respectful, but also egocentric and explosive. I had to vacillate between the two contrasting images of him on a daily basis. The effort to bring him into focus was re-wiring my brain. Small and commonplace functions were frustrating and infuriating for him. He took nothing in stride. I was always on call to sort out whatever mess he got himself into, whether it was finding something he misplaced, (naturally, he never misplaced anything, it was always someone else) or trying to repair something when its mechanics eluded him. As soon as I learned Clay couldn't change the oil in a car, I taught him how. For a year or so it seemed to go rather smoothly, until one Saturday afternoon he came into the house with a reddish fluid all over his hands. "What's on your hands?" I asked. "It's oil," he replied. Wait a minute I thought oil was amber when it's new and black when it's used. "Clay, that's not oil, it's transmission fluid." Clay's car had developed a metallic "ping" in the engine about two months before, and a picture began forming in my mind. Sure enough, Clay had been draining the transmission fluid and adding more oil. The engine block was baked in oil and the transmission case was as dry as a bone. That oil change cost $1200.00. I learned not to depend on Clay for mechanical repairs.

Clay was not a partner or a teammate. He never played sports, but could tell you anything you wanted or didn't want to know about the subject. We weren't a team, either. If he was washing up at the kitchen sink and I needed to rinse my hands under running water at the same time, he would back up across the room throw his hands up in the air; snarling and snorting as if I had insulted him. Something as benign as sharing space was difficult for him. Our efforts to work together were pathetic—an awkward ballet of mal-jointed dancers, bumping into each other, and grimacing at their partner's ineptitude.

We couldn't make up a bed together. Simple chores I had done many times with others were beyond his comprehension and ability. He lacked the natural rhythm and intuition needed when working with anyone, things like knowing when to hand over a screwdriver instead of wrench or when to grab the other end of something being moved.

He would require in-depth instruction and direction to accomplish the most elementary and common chores, I had to bite my tongue to keep from asking him, "And how long have you been on the planet"? Of course, he would be grumbling and arguing the fine points of how to accomplish anything whether he had done it before or not. I got to the point where it was much faster, though harder, to do things alone than to have to debate him.

Clay's knowledge came through reading rather than experience; published instructions became engraved in his head and were the only acceptable method to accomplish anything. He trusted the printed word over any personal experience or common sense I had. Clay thought he could do anything by simply reading about it, but he always ran into a problem with application. Once I asked him to help me hang a shower curtain rod. It was one of the spring-loaded expandable types. The label stated that it would fit a space 42" to 60", but he was determined it was too short and kept grabbing it away from me to return to the store, "Clay, you have to unscrew it to the desired length." He stood there with arms folded over his chest glaring at me until I was able to adjust and slide it into place. I should have done it alone. During the years when I was a single mother, I became independent and learned how to do many of my own home and car repairs, minor ones, at least, so I was quite surprised at how inept Clay was at doing any of these tasks.

His response to my requests for assistance was akin to me, a peasant, asking the royal head of the castle to jump in and lend a hand. When anyone commented on the repairs around the house, it seems we had done it. I assume it was the royal "we."

Clay was an authentic intellectual down to his delicately tapered fingertips. He did not putter around the house or the garage making repairs or organizing, and thankfully, he never fiddled with the cars again. When he was at home and not sleeping, eating or reading the only puttering he did was on his computer— this was my rival and his mistress.

## CHAPTER 8

*"The ship, a fragment detached from the earth, went on lonely and swift like a small planet."*
—Joseph Conrad

My girlfriends and I would get together and coffee klatch, less often since all of us had remarried. We relaxed and chatted about how our children were doing, how much weight had been lost and regained, and how content everyone was—until it was my turn. I sank back into my chair and with my best imitation of a casual attitude declared, "Oh, nothing much to tell." Liar! There was too much to tell.

They had allowed me to get away with no disclosure about my marriage for over two years, but this time they cornered me and refused to let up until I spilled the beans. They wanted to know why I had become such a recluse and when exactly did I lose my sense of humor and self-confidence. I was speechless—was it that obvious? Could people look at me and tell I had changed and was not aware of it? Actually, I thought I had artfully concealed my disappointment over my marriage. I never let it slip during a chance meeting or a telephone conversation I was anything but busy. Busy with work, the kids, the house. Even at dinner parties with Clay at my side, I wore a deceptive smile, while producing enough stomach acid to erode the bottom of a battleship. A sense of foreboding tagged along with us on any social occasion. Would he do or say something to confound and embarrass me? Yeah, boy! I was a lucky woman. I had the man of my dreams. I had the whole enchilada.

On this day, surrounded by friends, I realized my charade was transparent and useless under the keen scrutiny of these wise women. We knew each other too well, and any attempt on my part to hide anything from them was pure self-deception. We had been through heartbreak, cancer, cancer scares, injured children, marginal poverty and lots of coffee. We had shared it all, but never anything close to what I had lodged in my brain.

I must have in some frantic self-deluding moment made an internal pledge to keep this confusing, disorienting information to myself. If I didn't tell anyone, I would be free to believe that one day things would change through my diligent patience and dedication to the marriage. I was going to stubbornly apply CPR to this lifeless corpse of a relationship until it was resuscitated or someone pulled me away. In the meantime, I wouldn't suffer the humiliation of anyone knowing about my mind blowing state of matrimony. No one was going to see my tormented lonely existence and heap pity or judgment on me. I was in the unenviable position of having to decide which pain to bear—the pain inherent with keeping a dark secret and living with it in isolation, or the humiliation of people knowing I had failed at marriage—twice!

I had to wonder: who was I protecting, Clay or me? It wasn't a simple question. Complicated by pride and a sense of betrayal, I sensed that these raw issues weren't going to be solved by logic, conventional wisdom, or well-intended friends. It was loaded with painful consequences—the kind I wasn't prepared to accept. If I told them, would they lose respect for me for becoming a victim of emotional abuse or would they advise me to leave him? Would they understand I couldn't leave without knowing what was wrong, or how else would I avoid anything similar in the future? Of course the real hook was—suppose I could repair it. I was a first class sucker for closure and fixes.

I really didn't know what responses my story would elicit from them and it made me nervous being interrogated even by close friends. Bottom line: I wasn't confident that I could trust anyone with this very private, intimate information about Clay. I was afraid they would ask me questions I couldn't answer or would feel uneasy about answering. Did I want to blurt out, "Hey, girls, guess what? I made a monumental mistake and chose the wrong man, he's an imposter!" I could simply admit to a nice plump, ripened paranoia, and say I had been tricked, or more to the point—I had been duped into believing I was on the receiving end of a real catch. I could be bluntly honest, "Ladies, I was robbed!"

I also imagined telling them in a calm conversational tone that all the attributes I originally thought I saw in Clay were superficial. What I didn't see and assumed was present was an emotional structure which turned out to be smoke and mirrors. The mirror reflected only what I wished to see. I had projected all the desired qualities I wanted in a husband onto Clay. I was gagging on my reckless selection of a mate.

I was swallowing several gallons of angst everyday and wanted nothing more than to throw-up this copious gorge. There was no safe repository for this volume of self-recrimination, disillusionment, and disappointment, and it certainly wasn't going to be my friends.

All of this internal dialogue took place at warp speed. Over the last few months, my mind was perpetually stuck in high gear; ramping up at each new mind-bending discovery about Clay and forcing me to frantically search for explanations.

Finally, I was able to take a breath and was ready to face the music; my flighty mind slowed and taxied back to the kitchen table where expectant friends began unloading my baggage. I could sense they were confused and hurt over my long silence on the subject. Secrets were not something I felt comfortable transporting around, but I was becoming rather adept at it: collecting, storing, and fiercely protecting them. Sharing anything about Clay's strange proclivities felt disloyal. I had always been an open book to my friends and this newly acquired habit of hiding things was excruciatingly out of character for me.

They jumped right in and began probing for the trigger point.

Lynn gently began the inquisition. "What's going on with you? Are you okay?" Placing her hand on mine, "I mean it's not your health, is it?"

"No, I'm okay." I wanted to add that I was a nervous wreck, but that could cover anything from perimenopause, living with teenagers, or too much coffee.

Jean piped up, "Are the kids alright?"

"I'm taking Mark to therapy, but the girls are doing well." I told them about my son's problem, adding that his therapist told me she was happy with Mark's progress.

Bette anted up the first salvo. "How's Clay? Is he still working with computers?"

"Oh, yes."

"What do you two do for fun? Jim and I go the coast every time we get the chance. He wants to move down there when we retire."

"We just stay around here; Clay likes to read and I . . ." My answer trailed off and was left hanging unfinished and weighted.

An embarrassing silence fell around the table; I waited to regain control over the impulse to purge myself of my toxic cargo.

All eyes turned in my direction while spoons clinked against coffee mugs and fingers eagerly pinched stray crumbs from empty plates. I didn't know where or how to begin, so I began with tears—the universal language of distress. I wept as their loving concern touched me with their familiar nurture—a gentle comfort, which Clay denied me.

They sat patiently while I gutted a box of tissues. I blew my nose, wiped my face, and apologized over and over for breaking down. Finally, after I had shed enough water to make another pot of coffee, I told them about our pathetic love life—demands for details pelted me like a hard slanting rain. I cautiously began to relate the humiliating events that had taken place.

"He won't make love to me." I shrugged.

"What's wrong with him, is he impotent?"

"No, I don't think so. Everything seemed to be functioning okay when we had sex last year."

"Last year? Did you say last year?"

"Yes."

"Does he say why?"

"He won't talk about it."

"Oh, honey, mine doesn't like to talk either. Doesn't he know how this is upsetting you?"

"I guess not."

Lynn asked the next natural and expected question about any husband's aberrant behavior. "Is there someone else?"

"I don't think so, he's home every night and all weekend. If there is, I don't know when he would see her."

Bette had the nerve to ask what everyone was thinking—"Is he gay?"

"I don't think so, he subscribes to Playboy." I said it as if this was the definitive proof of male virility and sexual orientation.

"What do you think is wrong?"

"I don't know what to think, he's different from any man I have ever known. I've never had a man treat me this way."

Initially, they gave me their tender consolatory responses:

"Well, you just hang in there, maybe he just needs time."

"Men can be insensitive jerks, but I'm sure he loves you."

As I tried my best to describe the indescribable, they soon abandoned their genuine efforts to console me as my allegations outpaced their ability to interpret and justify Clay's actions.

Of course, I knew men could at times be insensitive, unromantic, or even downright stupid—we all knew that, but I also gave men in general more credit for being decent as well as victims of the same harsh judgments and misunderstandings as women. I had a view of people that was optimistic and hopeful. Surely, I believed, not all men were guilty of all of Clay's insensitive and hurtful behavior.

"Well, you need to see a therapist." It was a unanimous vote given by the nodding of heads. Problem solved. I would see another therapist who would, in a sterile clinical setting, remove my "Gordian Knot" and my life would make sense.

They had all assumed that since Clay was non-threatening (on the surface), a veritable "teddy bear" of a man, whatever the problem, they felt it was not beyond remedy. I blew my red swollen nose, gave an affirmative nod followed by a weak smile.

In my heart I knew they still didn't get it, but then neither did I.

When everyone stood up and prepared to leave, I was suddenly overcome with a sense of dread. I couldn't blame them for my long absences from our circle of sisters; I felt disconnected from their way of life, an outsider, and I was longing for the happiness I lost and they had. I was beginning to pull away and separate myself from the people I needed the most; those who brought a respite from my surreal life. On some gut level, I felt as long as I was with Clay I would never have a normal existence. Clay and happiness felt mutually exclusive.

Their presence filled the room with a light and warmth, which had been absent from my dismal existence far too long. We hugged good-bye with promises to do this again, real soon. I felt the life support slipping away and wanted cry out, "Take me with you!" I wanted to inhale their strength and contentment: a mixture compounded of oxygen and euphoria. I wanted to be one of them again. I wanted to feel happy and alive.

In their company I was in a freeze frame of sanity. A comfortable and life-affirming moment, which reminded me I, too, once lived in a vibrant world of warm, animated inhabitants who spoke a shared language. I knew once they left, my new courageous resolve to move in any constructive direction would wane and crumble as the coming days and weeks passed in the alternate universe where I resided. Where I had once been the strong one, the nurturing one, I was now the pitied one.

I was so angry with Clay. Wasn't this the purpose of a spouse to support each other spiritually and emotionally? Why wasn't he doing these things? I could feel the tiny fissure spreading rapidly through my heart and quickly filling with fury and rankle.

His neglect in so many sensitive areas had forced me into a life of shameful panhandling—"Will work for emotional support and validation."

It was nearly ten years before I met with my friends again; during that long interval, I did see quite a few therapists. My friends with their listening hearts were better healers. They didn't understand the conundrum at the center of my life, and couldn't give me any answers, but then none of us had known anyone like Clay.

They always left love on my doorstep, even when they had no entry. Our meeting that day brought home one new fear and attached itself to me—what if no one ever understood it?

## CHAPTER 9

*"There ain't no answer. There ain't going to be any answer. There never has been an answer. That's the answer."*

—Gertrude Stein

At the time, I wasn't aware that I was setting out into uncharted territory when I called on the mental health profession.

This was to be a journey of discovery, but the only discovery made apparent was that no one knew what in the world I was talking about.

I was not a person easily frustrated—only when trying to untangle Christmas tree lights or losing those last stubborn five pounds on a diet. Living with Clay put me in a state of terminal frustration and I managed to elevate this once fleeting emotion to the level of an art form replete with creative expletives.

An accurate analogy of my relationship with Clay would be the two of us on a tandem bicycle with me in the front peddling furiously and he in back with his feet off the peddles, legs stretched straight out, and yelling, "Whee!" I would have to face yet another fact: Clay was along for the ride and this was all I could ever expect of him. He displayed no interest in improving the marriage. I had tried hard to find the answer as to why, but I hit a brick wall at every turn. Whatever was at the core of his makeup taunted me daily and was close to pushing me over the edge.

Over a period of ten years, I visited several therapists; very quickly, I became discouraged.

First, I was frustrated by my lack of a lexicon suitable for describing Clay and, second, by their unwillingness to explore my grievances about Clay's enigmatic and infuriating personality.

One therapist after seeing us as a couple offered this little ditty as her counsel for our anemic sex life: "All cats are gray in the dark."

I had no idea what Clay took away from that session, but I personally don't allow cats in the bedroom.

Another therapist concluded after two sessions that Clay seemed non-threatening. His unstated but inferred counsel had a load of gender bias attached; I was just one more neurotic female who didn't understand or appreciate her man—precisely! One countered every complaint I had about Clay with anecdotes about her troubled history as an abused child. I handed her tissues until my hour was up. At the end of my session, she asked that I leave by the back exit; she was expecting a "high profile" client due to come in through her front entrance. I meekly followed her directive and slunk out to the parking lot feeling cast off and worthless. By now, the fight had been drained out of me and it was apparent in my lack of a reaction to her dismissive attitude.

How could I flunk therapy? I don't know, but somehow I managed to. Like a blind pilgrim to Lourdes, I had come to them in search of a miracle, but was sent away empty-handed.

I was convinced either Clay or I was short a few marbles, but all the evidence was beginning to lead to me.

Whenever Clay accompanied me to sessions, he sat quietly and answered questions articulately and politely.

"Why do you think your wife is depressed?"

"I don't know."

The therapist centered the focus on me because I was the only one miserable and willing to talk about it. Clay had no clue as to why I was upset even in the light of all my complaints.

The conversations between Clay and the therapist were so civilized and amicable and were carried on as though I wasn't in the room.

Clay gave the impression he was familiar with the subject of marital pitfalls and the subsequent remedies as if he had recently finished reading the textbook and passed the final exam. He could pass himself off to look much better with professionals than the reality I experienced with him at home.

I sat in the room thinking, why don't you have a fit for him, show him who you really are. Damn it, do something abnormal! I was screwed—no one would ever witness Clay's episodes that drove me into absolute despair.

What did happen only served to discourage me more. We were informed in couples' therapy that communication is the bedrock of a good marriage. Our therapist briefly explained the rules and described the tools used in therapy—a modality, which centered on perception and communication.

"Don't say, 'you', when discussing your problem and use, 'I feel'." Clay understood this, and given the parameters of communication with rules, he was on board 100%.

Rules facilitated Clay's social interactions. He loved rules—no second guesses, no need for personal judgments required, and most importantly, no gray areas, which would confuse him. He wouldn't be required to interpret facial expressions or body language—simple and straight forward. Piece of cake!

The therapist asked us to explain the problem. I began with my common complaint of no communication or intimacy. I began with the lack of a sex life, because I knew without a doubt that this was a concrete indication that something was off, way off. All my other complaints were rather hazy and could be considered delusional.

Clay morphed from the actively informed into the passively clueless.

"Clay, can you tell me what you think the problem is?"

"Well . . . what she said," he explained.

"Yes, but do you agree?" The therapist eased to the edge of his chair.

"I think so." At this rate, we would be the oldest couple in therapy history struggling with walkers into his office.

Looking at me again, the therapist asked me to continue.

"We haven't had sex in eight years and he won't talk about it."

"Clay, is this true?" Dr. Man shot me an incredulous expression.

"Yes." Clay looked down at the carpet and began sawing his index finger across his thumb (one of his quirky habits employed when he found himself the center of unwanted attention).

"If you both agree that this is a problem area, then I suggest we begin with this issue."

He was patient with Clay, whereas after years of his resistance to my questions, I would have throttled him.

"First, I need to ask if there is some physical basis for this hesitancy to engage in sexual intercourse. Clay, is everything functioning?"

"Yes." Highly uncomfortable, Clay looks away.

"So, can you tell me what you feel is the reason you aren't interested in engaging in sex with your wife?" Therapist eases back into his chair and steeples his hands in preparation for some profound disclosure from Clay.

"She says she can't tell when I want sex."

Eyes shift to me, the primary suspect.

"He never makes advances and he doesn't behave like a man who wants sex, and I got tired of asking him and getting rejected."

"Okay"; a gently rocking nod by therapist.

"Clay is that right?"

"I guess so."

Then Clay said something that not only shocked me, but also accorded me a key to a distant locked door.

"Sometimes, I feel like I am thirteen years old."

"Why do you feel like you're thirteen?"

"I don't know."

"Clay, sometimes we can feel like a helpless child, or when we feel a lack control in our lives"; an artless response left hanging in midair.

Then Dr. Man turned to me and explained, "If men are feeling pressured by stresses at work or at home, they can develop a sexual malaise or a diminished libido.

I was off in some faraway zone thinking about Clay's unprecedented statement; this unexpected revelation created a constriction in the pit of my stomach.

All at once, Clay came into full focus for the first time in all these years. Yes, he was thirteen years old. That was the gnawing feeling—the strange, mind-splitting image that lingered below the surface of his physical adulthood.

I snapped back into the moment to answer the last question, but I was no longer concentrating on the session; instead, I was mentally running through the past scenarios this startling epiphany brought to the table.

"Yes," I answered, "but from the beginning of the marriage and continuing for eight years, isn't that a little excessive?"

"Well, yes. However, solutions for this specific problem can't be forced."

I felt he was angry; he wrote in his notebook and didn't look at me.

Great! This was all, my fault—I alone was responsible for Clay's lack of desire. Hurt and humiliation seared through me in a hot jagged assault; tears welled up in my eyes. I felt he was handling Clay with cashmere mittens and jabbing at me with boxing gloves.

This is how it was and would always remain—Clay would always be given the benefit of the doubt regardless of how much pain I was in or how much I needed help.

Sent home to work on our communication skills and some simple exercises in intimacy, Clay looked eager to comply with these instructions, and approached them as if he could earn a grade; he was going for a 4.0. He just didn't get it. This was not an intellectual challenge; this was about relationships—with illogical, messy and immeasurable emotions. I knew we were doomed; I knew Clay well enough to know he would lose interest and spend all of our allotted time doing this exercise while repeating the damn rules. By the time our check cleared the bank we would be back at square one.

In the presence of professionals he was their equal, he could talk the talk. When we left, they all but congratulated me on my choice of a mate.

My little inner voice of eroding sanity cautioned me to smile politely, choke back the primal scream permanently nesting in my chest, walk out the door, go home, take a valium, lie down and face the one indisputable truth—I was the one who was nuts.

They all accepted Clay's tractable demeanor and used it as an indictment of my assumed departure from reality. No one would ever believe me and I would leave this world behind with "Cassandra Syndrome" scribbled in bold, black ink on my toe tag as a disreputable epithet.

The infuriating truth was apparent to me if no one else—if Clay had been an alcoholic, a drug addict, or had physically abused me, I would have been the fortunate recipient of support, empathy, and understanding while I sported black eyes and an arm cast—wounds of real suffering. Clay's manner of abusive neglect was an insidious form of emotional battering—my bruises were deep below the surface.

The mental health profession had effectively muted my testimony as a witness to Clay's disorder; in their defense this was the late '80s and early '90s. The DSM (Diagnostic and Statistical Manual for Mental Disorders) was missing the diagnostic criteria which would eventually explain Clay. No one suspected what it was; they had all failed to recognize this elusive and un-christened disorder, which could masquerade with chameleon-like ability as a dozen different disorders or, apparently, none.

I gave up my quest for answers from the mental health field and doggedly pursued a course of self-medication for my own self-diagnosis. I was neurotic or delusional, perhaps both.

I went to my doctor about various physical complaints and eventually began taking anti-depressants. I hated them; they changed me into a zombie—like Clay. I couldn't cry when I needed the release; I didn't feel like myself, which under the circumstances was probably a good thing since I was no longer, me.

I began going to massage therapists, manicurists, and hair salons—I was paying people to touch me. I felt shame and thought if Clay or his parents knew about it, they would perceive me as weak; touching appeared to be unimportant to them and they would probably consider it a nonessential narcotic for the feeble-minded.

I continued with my pursuit of innocent tactile pleasures. I felt the human touch was important to maintaining health, physically and emotionally. Eventually, I became unaccustomed to touch.

I was suffering from an emotional form of marasmus. I was wasting away in many quarters. I needed something to feed my withering soul. I was tired of feeling like some wretched animal backed into a dark cave, waiting to die.

I developed a weakened immune system and became a sponge for any invading bacteria or virus. It was progressively harder to bounce back from simple infections. My doctor was puzzled; tests revealed no medical explanation for it. He suggested I see a therapist. I became a human tennis ball, hammered back and forth between medical and mental health practitioners with no definitive results. Enough! I screamed to myself. This is your life, it's never going to get better, and it's never going to change; no one can fix it and no one cares!

One winter I was sick with the flu. I was running a temperature of 103 degrees and couldn't lift my head off the pillow. Clay stopped by my room on his way to work and waved good-bye saying, "Have a nice day." I had to call him later and tell him I was unable to drive myself to the doctor's office. Clay drove me. While the doctor attended me, Clay stayed in the room and told the doctor about all the new medical studies he recently read. When he began suggesting new treatments for me, I asked Clay, to the doctor's relief, to leave the room so I could hear my physician's instructions without Clay's irritating interruptions. Clay ignored the fact that I was the reason for the visit and it wasn't an opportunity to showcase his brilliance in the field of scientific research.

When it came to medical care, Clay was a royal pain-in-the-derrière. He called to make an appointment for his first colonoscopy, and the doctor's secretary told him after an hour of trying to schedule the procedure he was a "nit-picker" and to call someone else. I had to smile when he related the incident; granted it was a small victory, but at last, I wasn't the only one who got his potential to be a major pain.

Clay rarely got sick; he sailed through life unaffected by ailments of the body and mind suffered by the majority of humanity. He had a particularly eerie immunity to emotional disorders. He never exhibited any signs of depression, disappointment, sadness, indecision, grief or despondency and why should he, I was handling all of those negative emotions for the both of us. On the other hand, he didn't show any of the positives: joy, happiness, elation, anticipation, spontaneity, spirituality, affection, humor or imagination. I thought a brain scan would show a fat, squatty, and contented little mushroom perched inside his cranium.

Once in a while I would skim though pages of personality disorders to satisfy myself I had exhausted every possible avenue of explanation for Clay's upsetting and befuddling actions in the off chance I had missed something. It was the same old maze, with me as the crazed rat searching for the elusive cheese. At least I had one promising clue and it would eventually facilitate the process of unraveling this daunting puzzle.

THE AARDVARK'S WIFE

## CHAPTER 10

*"I would rather believe God did not exist than believe that He was indifferent."*
— George Sand

As my social circle shrank to the circumference of a contracted pupil, and my children took a firm grasp on their adult lives, I had to acknowledge the inevitable—I would soon be living alone with Clay.

Rather than planning for my escape from this marriage, I had used my financial resources for my children's education, their weddings and domestic launchings. It was with an enormous sense of ambivalence that I released them from my arms and home—I would miss them terribly.

Their presence at home helped to maintain an optimistic outlook over the years, confident there would be hugs with sweetly uttered endearments, emotional rewards, and voices with modulated intonations coming and going on a daily basis.

I watched wearing a brave smile while my son, the last to leave, and his new bride carried out the remainder of his belongings from his childhood home. I mistakenly thought I was prepared for the day when I would no longer be a resident parent—it felt far different from what I had expected.

After they drove away, I went upstairs to his vacated room; it looked as huge as the hole in my heart felt. I began picking up the scattered debris left behind by his haphazard method of packing that was as familiar a signature as his handwriting. I spotted an old ratty shoelace from a long ago discarded sneaker; I picked it up and wound it into a small ball and stuck it in my pocket. That night while undressing, it fell to the floor—a soft, tangible reminder of his occupancy in our home. I walked to the waste basket next to my bed and let it fall from my hand. It wasn't the first, nor would it be the last time I would cut a cord.

My son moved out when he went away to college and then again when he joined the service, but this time I knew he wouldn't be back. He was a grown man with a wife and my job was done.

I knew my children would come for the holidays and would continue to include me in their busy new lives, but their absence resounded in every room of the house with a painful truth echoing all around me—I was alone in a way I had never anticipated. The walls would no longer reverberate with my children's unconstrained laughter and the celebrations that accompanied their successes, or reflect the soft sounds of tears following failure and heartbreak, the latter allowing me to embrace and comfort them. I would miss my family who showed expressions of happiness as well as sadness, whose faces told me of their inner feelings and who, unlike Clay, could read mine and would offer the appropriate response. Small gestures I had been allowed to take for granted and gave me so much comfort.

Without the frenetic pace of a household of young adults who brought me a welcomed diversion from my torpid existence with Clay, my life decelerated from eighty to zero.

The knowledge I was not a wife in any traditional sense was exacerbated by a depressing epiphany—I was also childless.

I began to work longer hours to avoid going home and facing the nothingness that Clay offered. Instead of looking forward to my new freedom from parental obligations or feeling a new lightness of spirit—I felt lost and restless. I couldn't look forward to a second honeymoon like so many of the couples in our age group. We had no love life; this in itself was not conducive to romantic fantasies. This was supposed to be the beginning of a new chapter in my life; however, it felt like an ending. I wondered what my future would be with only Clay. His ideal retirement plan was to re-read the hundreds of science fiction and fantasy books he owned. His books took up so much space. I thought it would be highly economical if someone could make edible books; if they could be consumed twice, it would save room and groceries. Second on his list was sleeping. Thankfully, I was years away from that gloomy prospect.

The only thing I could do to insure any future happiness would be to plan for my financial independence and then leave. But at the same time, I really didn't want to abandon the hope that one day Clay might include me in his life as something other than a roommate. It was extremely difficult to plan my life while vacillating between finding a reason to stay and feeling the need to leave.

Clay didn't say much about the children after they moved out, but he did seem to be affected by Mark's departure. He always wanted my son to share his interests, but chess and reading were sedentary and boring to a teenager. Mark tried to find some common interest to please Clay, but he was too active and athletic to sit still long enough to acquire any patience for Clay's interests. Over the years, the kids referred to him as the "Nerd" or the "Geek" because of these particular preoccupations and his inability to converse in any area outside of dry statistical data.

Mark was disappointed when his stepfather wouldn't participate in sports—Clay had a clumsy gait and poor hand-eye coordination. He had a hard time catching a baseball, or even car keys (his fingers, with the exception of when he was having a fit and spreading them, were rigid and stayed in a tight, frozen alignment whenever he tried to catch objects), but he was actually an excellent bowler. The one thing that Clay excelled in was sport statistics and game rules. He usually attended sports events with me when my children were playing. He enjoyed the games, but never complimented them on their accomplishments.

Occasionally, I detected sadness in Clay after Mark left; it occurred to me Clay felt a loss, not for a son, but rather a playmate or perhaps a sibling. It was unusual for a man to miss a grown stepson more than his wife's companionship.

Given the new circumstance I found myself and my diminished social outlets, I tried, again, to draw Clay into some semblance of a relationship. When I wasn't the lone student in an isolated lecture hall being tutored by Mr. Spock about the essential use of logic and unlimited amounts of information in general, I would try to draw Clay into discussions about some of my interests. I thought we should be able to find some mutual ground to use as a foundation for building a new deeper understanding and tolerance for each other's passions.

I began a conversation (which quickly became a debate) about the creation of the universe and the earth. He jumped right to the Big Bang theory, and I countered with the Creationist theory. Naturally, I was stupid to believe such a far fetched concept! Of all the ridiculous thoughts a human could have, this was the most compelling argument for man's inability to evolve intellectually. Who could possibly believe in a fairy tale perpetuated by theologians for millennia in the face of the mountains of physical and scientific evidence to the contrary? But I wasn't sure it was an antithesis; why couldn't a higher power such as God, who created the universe and the physical world, also create evolution? I could even accept the premise that it wouldn't follow the same order or timeline as described in the Book of Genesis, but I didn't have a problem believing that a supreme being was responsible. We believe we know how the big bang occurred from a purely astrophysical perspective, but we have to wonder: what was the catalyst that turned a gaseous chaos into a well-ordered universe? What came before?

The debate escalated from there while Clay tried to sway me with purely logical arguments, which I could accept up to a point, but suddenly, without fanfare or preamble, he hit one out of the park—he didn't believe there was a God. My mouth dropped open; I was unable to absorb the statement silently bouncing off the walls. To date, I thought I had discovered all the surprises Clay had to offer, but this one was as shattering as any he had hit me with in the past.

My mind scrambled to collect all the supporting evidence to the contrary: we attended church; he was raised by parents who took him to Sunday school every week and said Grace before meals. They knew the Bible in its entirety.

How could I have missed so much in a person who was as proximal as a spouse? This wasn't just an insignificant gap separating us, but an abyss of ignorance concerning the very essence that defined who we were.

I asked Clay why he never told me this when we were dating or since. "You didn't ask." So this was the deal: if I didn't ask, he wasn't going to be forthcoming. He would coast through life using the sin of omission as a get-out-of-jail-free pass. I was up to my ears in false assumptions about Clay, and I had no idea as to how many more were insidiously waiting to bite me in the behind.

I had seen positive traits in Clay: his kindness to animals and children and his morality, which up until now I believed emanated from a spiritual source. I would have to re-examine previous conjecture and admit that his morality was secular in nature—it came from following a rigid set of social and civil edicts.

Like his parents, Clay was a good citizen; they paid their bills and taxes and tithed to the church and voted. But, I had to wonder if these things alone made you a "good" person. I believed in service to others: the extending of oneself to those in need of comfort, food or spiritual support. They stopped short at reaching out to their fellow man or community. I didn't want to judge them; God knows, I am about as imperfect as it gets, but I was trying to understand how they could present themselves as Christians in the community without a core of spirituality. I am not talking about hypocrisy, but rather a dryness of the soul. The words and the music didn't go together.

When Clay and I joined our church, we and eight other couples met with our pastor. He moved around his small study and stood in front of each couple asking us individually our reason for becoming a member of his congregation. When it was our turn, Clay slipped between me and a bookcase, like a child hiding from a bully, sending shelves of books crashing to the floor. I was embarrassed by a grown man trying to slide his 6'2", 300lb frame behind me, as though he could hide behind anything smaller than a wooly mammoth. I stated my reasons for membership and Clay, who normally would launch into a long academic discourse on any subject, simply replied, "Me too."

When Clay amazed me with the revelation about his atheism, I couldn't help but wonder, how could I have fallen in love with someone who didn't believe in God? Why couldn't I see it? Clay, in spite of his intelligence and quasi-sophistication, had a naiveté and innocence about him, a childlike acceptance—I must have taken this as evidence of faith.

Clay and his parents had a far greater devotion and loyalty to science than to religion. I would go so far as to say it is their religion.

In any question regarding the physical world or humanity—science is always the correct answer.

While I rubbed my eyes in a futile effort to make the moment clearer, I realized I also assumed since Clay and his parents are so knowledgeable about the Bible, they were also disciples of its central tenet.

Clay's defense for a lack of faith went, "How can there be a God when there is so much suffering in the world?" He immediately became quiet with the expectation I would produce a glowing, shimmering celestial entity who could hurl lightning bolts across the room and incinerate the couch in order to reveal his divinity, personally, to Clay.

I told him I believed it's mankind with its inherent greed and selfishness who creates the suffering in the world, not God.

I had only my faith to counter Clay's disbelief. I believe in God and know we must come by faith alone. I couldn't give Clay the indisputable scientific proof he needed in order to become a believer. He would have to find it for himself and I prayed that he would.

Clay's statement reminded me of a quote from George Santayana: "The Bible is literature, not dogma." I concluded: the Bible's singular appeal to Clay—another source of information. He could use this sacred text as another opportunity to showcase his authoritative intellect. For him faith and intellect were conflicting values.

After learning about his disorder, I understood why Clay couldn't believe in God—he was only able to recognize and process values which were measurable and quantitative—and God was the ultimate abstract. He believed in the plausibility of extraterrestrials, but the great I AM would be the ultimate quantum leap.

# CHAPTER 11

*"We are so fond of one another, because our ailments are the same."*

—Jonathan Swift

Other than Clay's vague mention of his parents: "I ate dinner at my parents," or "I stopped by my parents to pick up my laundry," I hadn't met them although we all lived in the same town. He was living in his townhouse or rather, he was bathing, dressing and sleeping there; outside of the twice monthly cleaning service, his parents met his other domestic needs.

It was over a month after he had proposed before he felt it necessary to introduce me to my prospective in-laws. I don't know whose idea it was, his or his parents, but instead of an invitation to dinner to meet the folks, which is the usual custom, they were to come visit me at my home, on a Saturday afternoon. What horrible timing; weekends were chaotic with errands, laundry, my kids and their friends galloping through the house and leaving trails of teenage debris everywhere. I was unprepared for this interview-style of introduction and the subsequent inspection of my home and children.

I proudly introduced my children to Ben and Ellen and gave a brief bio of each one: name, age, scholastic achievements and capacity for bedlam. I gave a description of my job, shared some details about my social life and interests, and told them how much I enjoyed being with their son. No response. His father kept interjecting Clay's SAT scores into the conversation, which was strange and struck me as shameless promotion. It became clear they felt Clay's most sterling quality was his intellect. I chose to ignore it, believing Clay had greater potential as a husband than mere cerebral output.

The meeting felt awkward, as these things usually do. It had all the earmarks of an adoption interview between the natural parents and the prospective parent. I wasn't certain when it was over, if I was marrying or adopting him. I had looked forward to a perfunctory introduction and possibly some embarrassing stories from Clay's childhood, or some humorous family anecdotes; nope, just the SAT scores. This was my first trip down the Rabbit Hole and I would become a frequent guest.

Clay's parents were extremely intelligent people. His father held a PHD in Parasitology. The CDC considered him an international authority on the subject of parasites. He was the director of the Department of Public Health's laboratories in our state. He also taught at the School of Public Health at a local university. His mother had a degree in Chemistry and a minor in Home Economics. They met when Ellen went to work in the lab he managed, and after their wedding she never worked outside the home. They married six months after Ben's first wife died. These were smart people who were grounded in the hard sciences. I found them fascinating to listen to—at first. I was impressed by their knowledge and simultaneously puzzled by their family dynamic.

They were a quiet, well-ordered family. Their dinner conversations while interesting and somewhat stimulating were strangely devoid of familiarity. There were no inside jokes, laughter, or good-natured teasing, just serious conversations about new scientific studies. I would listen and watch as I searched for some common ground. Once, I offered a humorous take on one of the topics they had been chewing on all evening and their response was dead silence. They looked at me as though I had just sprayed Ebola over the dinner table.

They were not pretentious people and had standard etiquette at the dinner table; however, they had an irritating habit: they all spoke at the same time. I was amazed no one seemed to be listening but me. I was watching a frantic horserace. They were out of the gate and jockeying for first position, suspense rode every turn around the track, who would win? This was not a good natured and highly spirited conversation but a highly competitive debate, each one attempting to grab the coveted trophy—the last word. The loser would sit on the sideline and interject contradictions and asides in an attempt to regain lost status.

Family dinners consisted of the many delicious southern recipes I truly loved. Clay's mother was a good cook and took pride in providing meals that were nutritionally balanced, but terrifyingly fattening. I overindulged with seconds and desserts (there was always more than one dessert). I came to welcome the carbohydrate induced euphoria, which made the whole family-dinner raucous slightly more palatable for me. Some situations require drugs: childbirth and Clay's family dinners.

If I tried to join the verbal melee, I was usually ignored or drowned out. Finally, in frustration, I gave up. I remained silent and resigned to my place on the periphery of the table and the family. I concentrated on the plate in front of me while a convergence of discordant voices rose in a cacophony around me. Clay's mother would occasionally stop long enough to take a breath and ask me why I wasn't talking, but before I could answer she was on to another subject. This woman could talk and I mean talk. Forget about getting a word in edgewise; either she didn't think anyone else had anything of interest to offer, or she was the only one with anything important to say—I couldn't decide which. I do know, I was never allowed to make a statement, without Ellen contradicting, correcting or negating any and every word I said. Clay had this irritating habit, too. I learned the definition of a toxic person is someone who can't allow anyone else to be right. They certainly exemplified the word. I wouldn't be surprised if Webster's lists their names under the definition of toxic.

I always offered to help in the kitchen after dinner, thinking it a good opportunity to get to know her better, but she declined my help. She, too, had this fanatical need to arrange dishes in the dishwasher just so—that's when I understood where Clay got it from and had to smile. I wanted to use the time in the kitchen, out of earshot of Ben and Clay, to ask Ellen what caused Clay's episodic outbursts. When I was able to I ask, she shrugged and claimed she didn't know. Surprisingly, she wasn't in the least upset or curious about his behavior or what may have provoked it. Ellen and Ben, both, had been present during these disruptive displays on several occasions. They never said anything, but waited it out (making me think this was not new behavior and it was expected) and then resumed their conversations as if they had watched an ant wander across the table.

I felt unwelcome as a daughter-in-law. Clay's mother, Ellen, constantly brought up Clay's ex as if she was still an active member of the family. Sharon had remarried, but Ellen made it clear that she was still her daughter-in-law. "She is Melinda's mother." It was said with the same reverence as, "She is the holy Mother." I had no such genetic offering. She didn't consider how this might make me feel even more of an outsider.

She, like Clay, had an imperious air and never weighed her words or considered anyone's feelings in her straight forward and insensitive statements.

When Clay and I went to visit Ellen for Mother's Day, Easter or her birthday, Sharon was always there first. I was left in the car like the family dog while Clay went in and played family, sometimes leaving me for an hour or more. He never apologized for this deliberate exclusion; it was as if he couldn't see how uncomfortable this whole situation made me. He would come out to the car smiling and telling me what his mother served for lunch. Whatta guy!

Ellen did confide to me that his ex complained about him always having his nose in a book, and I could relate to that. She also told me that when they were married, Sharon said "mean" things about Clay that hurt her feelings. Hmm, maybe that marriage wasn't as perfect as Clay had led me to believe, and he was also clueless and blameless as to what had precipitated their divorce.

Although Clay's father, Ben, was closely associated with the medical community, he resented it for not recognizing his doctorate as the equivalent of a medical degree. He wrote his doctoral dissertation in German. I was impressed with his ability to understand a foreign language fluently enough to write a scientific thesis. He felt he was smarter than many medical doctors. This was a common diatribe at dinner.

None of them went for annual physicals. It appeared rather contrary to dislike a profession to the detriment of an individual's health and well-being. They thought it strange that I would go for regular check-ups. Clay would tell them I had gone to the doctor and they would ask if I was sick. "No, she just went for a check-up." "Well, why did she do that?" I was able, years later, to convince them to go for wellness visits. Ellen had a suspicious lump removed from her breast. I was relieved I was able to persuade her to go.

I began a campaign of reminding and even nagging to get them to take care of their health. Over time, I came to fill the role in their lives of a guardian.

On the surface, Clay and his parents impressed me as being stable people, living a well-ordered life. They lived by calendars and clocks with the predictability of circadian cycles. Birthdays, holidays and anniversaries were celebrated over Ellen's home cooked dinners. Guests included all of Clay's aunts and uncles, and Ellen's college roommate. These were the same guests at Melinda's birthday—no children her age, just adults. Ben had eight siblings, Ellen had one, a sister who lived out of state and visited three or four times a year. It did seem strange to me that in the forty-five years of their marriage, they had cultivated no "new" friends.

They made good neighbors; they kept the yard, the house and themselves in order and lived quietly and frugally. Their lifestyle was based on the "rules": the rules learned from the Bible, the social rules governing those interactions and of course, "good citizen" rules. It was all so perfect, so suspiciously ideal. The rules dictated their behavior and they expected everyone else to do the same. Anyone outside of Mother Teresa would come up short in the presence of this family and I was no exception. They were decent people living what appeared on the surface, a perfect existence. But they lacked some emotional qualities: spontaneity, joy and spirit. I often thought that this metered, safe life was stifling to the soul. A long road of "same ole, same ole" struck me as a soul-sucking routine defining their comfort zone. To me it looked as if they were walking a tightrope and any disturbance in the atmosphere would topple them over into a pit of absolute confusion.

When an emergency arose all the education and intelligence went out the window. They would begin what I called "trilling":

their voices would climb in desperate decibels, as they floundered for direction. I went through this with Clay and Ellen when Ben died. They would need someone to look after them, to make plans and interpret actions too subtle to comprehend or process. Even as this help was being executed they would remain imperious and contrary.

I cried when Ben passed and looked to Clay and his mother for the recognition in their eyes of a shared grief—there wasn't any.

There were many strange things in this family that I couldn't wrap my mind around. His dad was a kind man and I enjoyed talking with him. He loved his son and wife and it was evident in all he did. Ellen was a most unusual mother. At times, I perceived her as detached from nurturing as a mother in the wild who would disconnect the runt and leave it to perish. I could see her raising her two boys to fill the role in her life as little, adult companions, whom she would instruct in science and the rules. She didn't treat Clay like a son, but rather like another adult she didn't have any greater connection to than mutual interests. Ellen was not a woman who invited intimate discussions about personal issues and if I brought it up, she didn't offer any emotional support or comfort. She was pragmatic in her advice and delivered her counsel in much the same manner as Mr. Spock. The only warmth in her home came from the oven.

Clay had a younger brother, John, who died at the age of fifteen. He had a bone disorder that prevented the normal growth of this spinal column. In place of new bone growing on the outside of his spine, it grew in the interior of his vertebrae, eventually constricting his spinal cord. In gym class, while trying to execute a forward roll, his neck broke.

Clay's father cried when he told the story of John's death. Clay's mother said very little about him or his death and this concerned me. I asked Clay how his brother's death affected him. He shrugged his shoulders and said, "Dad didn't want us to talk about it because it might upset mother." "Yes, Clay, I understand that, but how did you feel? Were you sad, angry, or numb?" He didn't answer. I think it was a first for Clay, no one ever asked him how he felt about losing his only sibling. Sad.

Clay and his family didn't make mistakes or they didn't own up to any. Their lives and actions were calculated to the least degree of risk. Errors and missteps were the products of pitifully inferior minds. Mistakes require apologies, amends or facing fallibilities or more disastrously—culpability. All of these would require some measure of change in their method of thinking. They were survivalists—people who put their faith in their ability to reason, outsmart nature and their fellow man, and accumulate the necessary goods to insure their safety and security. They believed in science this gave them a measure of control over the physical world. They wouldn't share with their neighbors during a holocaust.

His mother's style of mothering was very basic: feed, clothe and educate; anything she couldn't do she would hire a tutor or offer a book on the subject. Clay told me his parents never had the "Talk" with him, but laid a book about sex on his bed.

No wonder having sex with Clay felt as if it came out of a manual—technical and unemotional.

She managed to feed Clay and Ben into obesity. His father became so heavy his legs wouldn't support his weight. When I suggested we take him to an indoor pool for exercise, she refused, saying "Oh, no, it's too much trouble."

"Ellen, we really don't mind, and it will help him with mobility and circulation," I pleaded.

"No, it's too much trouble," she re-iterated. Too much trouble for whom, I wondered. That was the end of the discussion.

Within a few months, he became sedentary and house bound. Restricted to a wheelchair, his health declined and he began having transient ischemic attacks. He was hospitalized and the day before he died, Clay, his mother and I visited him. I stood by his bed and held his hand; he looked at me and whispered, "Please take care of Ellen for me." I promised I would. Later, I thought the whole scenario was strange. Clay was in the room. Was not this a son's obligation to care for his surviving parent? I realized later that his father suspected Clay would be incapable of anticipating any need his mother may have in the future. I was correct.

Clay couldn't see when anyone, child or adult, was in trouble and needed help and evidently his mother couldn't either.

Amazingly, his parents, who had professional access to members of the medical community, since his father worked with doctors on a daily basis, never pursued a diagnosis for his brother's disorder. The post-mortem revealed John's condition. The impression I got was that this child's death came as a total surprise, and according to them, he showed no manifestations of a fatal condition. Clay explained that his brother's hands were malformed causing him to hold his pencil with a fist rather than his fingers. I couldn't believe that even in the mid-sixties with x-ray and other diagnostic tools, doctors couldn't detect a bone problem in John, assuming, he received any medical attention at all. There was something incongruous about an educated, science-savvy mother who wouldn't pursue a medical diagnosis for her child or even detect a condition that was potentially crippling or fatal.

I recall when Ellen's only sibling, an older sister, was in the hospital dying and she went out of state to visit her. I called to ask about Clay's aunt and how Ellen was holding up. Ellen's chilling response: "I wish if she's going to die anyway, she would hurry up and do it, so I won't miss my trip to Canada."

Cold and pragmatic, that's Ellen. Even when in the presence of her adored granddaughter, she didn't hug, kiss or fuss over her like most doting grandmothers. Ellen was not promiscuous with her feelings. Her approach to Melinda was of a custodial nature. Demonstrations of affection were missing. I eventually was able to encourage hugs in the family by greeting each of them with a big bear hug. Whether they enjoyed it or not, I'm not sure, but it made me feel better. If I wanted a hug from Clay, I had to ask for it, it wasn't something he did unsolicited.

Ellen and Ben treated Clay and Melinda like siblings, making certain if they gave one a gift, the other would receive something of equal value. On the occasion of Melinda's sixteenth birthday, her mother presented her with a brand new pick-up truck. Two days later, Ben and Ellen were at my office offering to buy Clay a pick-up truck because Melinda had one. With his hand poised over his checkbook, Ben asked how much it would cost. I was flabbergasted. I told them Clay didn't need a new truck, his car was less than three years old and he seemed quite happy with it. Granted it was a generous offer, but I wondered why he didn't go to Clay with this offer. Was I the assumed parental figure in Clay's life? Was the offer of a truck out of fear of a tantrum from Clay? It was bizarre and I never heard of it except in cases of sibling rivalry. It would be understandable in the case of Clay and John. Clay wasn't Melinda's sibling, he was her father. It also made me think that they used money in place of emotional support—giving gifts was a substitution for affection.

Although at times they could wander off base. The first Christmas, after Clay and I married, he asked what I would like for a gift. I told Clay I didn't really need anything, but for future reference, I did like handmade furniture. I can't describe how surprised I was when his parents presented me with a brand new power tool—a wood router, whatever that is.

They represented all the manifest indications of a well-educated, middle-class suburban family. Their intelligence was worrisome in the light of what looked like willful neglect of a young son's well-being. I sensed that something darker belied this idealistic image.

## CHAPTER 12

*"You start out with one thing, end up with another, and nothing's like it used to be, not even the future."*
—Rita Dove

It was the winter of 1997 and my mother and I were sitting in the somber waiting room of her oncologist. There were six others waiting. Some were perusing ancient magazines with little interest; one middle-aged woman knitted and occasionally patted the hand of the older man sitting beside her, probably her father, I thought. There was the recycled stale air of hope and hopelessness fused with equally stale piped-in music—it wasn't soothing or inspirational—over the next hundred years it would continue to play the same bland, staccato loop. The room's occupants exchanged quick nervous sound bites, fearful any lengthy conversations could tip the delicate scales weighted with optimism and dread. We sat still in the thin atmosphere we sucked in with shallow guarded breaths as we braced for death sentences.

During our visits over the next few months, we saw some new faces and fewer of the familiar ones. We never knew if an absence was good or terrible.

Mother was diagnosed with cancer and we spent the remainder of the spring and summer of that year with chemo, radiation and hospitalizations. During the short periods when she was able to stay home, we were enmeshed with feeding tubes, chemo med-lines and dosing schedules. Through it all I was her cheerleader, "We're gonna beat this!" I tried to rally her resolve and strength to keep fighting with my fragile waning belief that we would ever beat this horrible disease. In August, we received the dreaded news—we had a mere six weeks, plus or minus, to reconcile and prepare to say our good-byes—such a pitifully, short time to pack and unpack so much history, but I was and am thankful for it. Respectful of her wishes, I brought her home. My children and I kept a courageous and loving vigil as we witnessed my mother pass onto her next journey. My father was fatally wounded during World War II. My stepfather died in 1992. I became an orphan—in more ways than a human should be.

Mother's death was the catalyst for what would become the worst period of my life. I lost eight more souls over a twelve month span. I lost friends and relatives. They all left suddenly without good-byes. I lost the people whom I loved and loved me, the ones I turned to when my life with Clay became intolerable. They made me laugh, restored hope, and tendered encouragement for the times when I could only see despair.

As the death toll mounted, I had less time to grieve individually for anyone in the manner they deserved. Clay said he was sorry when I announced the death of yet another friend or relative and for one long year I went to funerals alone. I closed my business for good and allowed a heavy, black curtain to float down and envelop me. Death had obliterated my entire support network, and was surreptitiously making a reservation for me in limbo. Pinned under the suffocating weight of grief, I turned to Clay for support and comfort, but he showed no concern for me or the toll these losses were beginning to take on me.

After my mother passed, in the dark early hours before dawn, her body was taken away and my exhausted children left. Clay slept while mother died. I climbed the stairs, entered the bedroom and stood over him; I wanted to fall into his arms and feel the protection and comfort of my husband's arms around me—a homecoming with a sense of belonging. I shook him awake and, sobbed out, "My mother's gone, Clay." He awoke briefly and said, "I'm sorry." He turned over and went back to sleep. I lay on my side of the bed and wrapped by arms around a soaked pillow, I clung to it the remainder of the night letting my tears run freely and silently.

## THE AARDVARK'S WIFE

The next day his mother, Ellen, gave me the same austere, "I'm sorry." I had once before looked into their faces and searched for some meager recognition of the pain for the loss of a loved one when Ben passed, and now saw the same nothingness in their eyes, the same, familiar stoic resignation. I saw people who existed outside the main stream culture I embraced, but because they were so intelligent, I again, allowed this quality to make me doubt my core values and beliefs. I actually thought Ellen, the faithful church member and biblical expert would embrace me and my loss by saying, "Dear, try to remember, she's out of pain and in a better place." Aside from asking my husband for a hug, which was delivered in the same everyday manner as helping me with my coat, that was it. It seems regardless of how minute my expectations, they were capable of disappointing me in any given situation. Whenever, there was an occasion which demanded an emotional response to someone's misfortune, Clay, his mother and daughter would utter the same banal condolence, "I'm sorry." They all studied the same book of rules, when something bad happens, say you're sorry—one size fits all.

I don't recall much from this period of interminable mourning except for brief moments of clarity when I became aware of complete isolation. I don't recall eating, but I must have although I did lose twenty pounds—somehow. I don't remember anyone coming or calling. I remember Clay, the stoic, and Clay, the remote.

As I run the footage of this painful memory in reverse, I see him as a ghost figure silently pursuing his daily routine and never showing the slightest concern as I disappeared a little more each day.

He was as disinterested and disconnected in these traumatic moments of my life as any other I experienced. Clay had managed to irrevocably redefine the terms: husband and marriage. I needed him to shelter me, to tell me it was going to be alright and support my recovery. His irresponsible neglect and detachment served to hasten my descent into the most painful, soul wrenching cubicle available in hell—total isolation.

For several months, I passed the time in the fetal position on the floor of the family room trying to hang on to the edge of the universe while I grieved for those I loved and missed. My close friends, Jean and Frank, died within months of each other. They were the only couple I knew who could tolerate Clay's odd behavior and need to monopolize each and every conversation. They always raved about my cooking, which Clay never did, and they made me feel good and valued as a friend, they offered validation to a starved ego. My ex's mother died a few months later, burdening my children with grief for both their beloved grandmothers. I grieved for her too, for the value she represented in my children's lives. My friend, Gates, a close confidant for over thirty years, died unexpectedly from a massive heart attack three days before we were to meet for lunch. Two cousins who were close and very dear to me died following the others within months, and then before I could hang up my funereal attire, my Aunt Libby who was also my Godmother died and her passing was the final blow separating me from my depopulated world.

Night after night Clay came home from work, stepped over me and asked no one in particular, "What's for dinner." I became unmoored, free floating in a lifeless place without sound, light, or succor—submerged in a deprivation tank—a dark, warm womb where I closed my eyes and drifted off into the vastness of my new abode and ignored him. Whenever I opened my eyes he was in his chair reading not in the least aware or concerned that I was disappearing and might never return.

I was beyond pity. I was beyond self-pity. Clay seemed to feel no sense of urgency in reclaiming me. He didn't know there was something terribly wrong. Did he compare me to a wounded animal kicked to the side of the road after an accident and beyond salvage? I think Clay never understood the danger or damage from grief or depression.

One day my eldest daughter called; she had not seen me in the months following my mother's death, but she heard the disturbing specter of surrender in my voice. She called Clay at work and told him to take me to a doctor and get help. It had to take someone else to convince him I was in deep trouble. He prided himself on his vast knowledge of everything, but he saw nothing, especially me, vanishing by degrees right under his nose.

I sat in a psychiatrist's office while Clay read outside in the waiting room of the local Looney Bin.

The doctor spoke to me calmly and asked: "Were you sexually molested as a child?"

"No."

"Have you ever tried to kill yourself?"

"No."

I don't remember what else we talked about or why I wasn't committed or had no additional therapy, probably because Clay couldn't or wouldn't give him an accurate picture of what was going on at home. I learned from my past therapy sessions not to mention any problems with Clay. I took the path of least resistance—I accepted his diagnosis of depression and grief. After living with Clay they were familiar companions.

Medication was prescribed and coupled with Clay's ongoing neglect these became the management tools for a mundane textbook condition.

Once again oblivion called and I opened the leaden door and crawled through. The pleasures of suspended animation awaited me; I was grateful to be home alone, without another human presence—this was the assurance I needed to prevent the cravings of comfort and support a fractured spirit requires from another, from those who were never coming. Clay's presence was a psyche tease, physically present but inaccessible and unaware of another's suffering.

Clocks and calendars were of no interest to me I had nowhere to go and no travel companion. Day and night shed their delineation, months came and went dragging the seasons past my window unobserved and uncelebrated. I was in an existential default —eat, eliminate, sleep, and repeat. I was drifting past planets, clouds of cosmic dust, and time; this silent world for the untethered had only one inhabitant—me. Even God would have to search for me and I couldn't name one reason why He or anyone else should.

I sank deeper into the warmth and security of my pharmaceutically enhanced cocoon teetering on a precipice above a chasm of despair. For one year, I stayed in the room where my mother died, and wanted to do the same.

Without warning, a primordial imperative buried within me roused, triggered by either a benevolent life force or my medication wearing off, I don't know, but I sensed a powerful energy determined to exact me from the depths of unconscious surrender.

I felt a seed of survival stretching toward the light, and I wanted to come back, not to a life with Clay's selfish and neglectful actions which contributed to a life robbing depression. But, I wanted to see my children and grandchildren, I came back for them.

I began with small, life affirming steps. I began going back to massage therapy and my massage therapist concerned about my shaky emotional state referred me to a counselor who helped restore me and reintroduced me to optimism.

I was a blubbering lump of humanity as I sat across from her while I sobbed out the events of the last two years. After fifteen minutes of evaluation, she was confident I had PTSD (post traumatic stress disorder). I cried some more, but this time it was from relief. I had something real, something recognizable by the mental health profession and I hoped, treatable.

Grace Rowlson had training in the conventional methods of therapy and was the quintessential therapist, a professional, but possessed a valuable attribute few in her field possessed—she was spiritually gifted. I felt safe and unafraid to open up and share with her my darkest fears and secrets. She understood why I didn't want to take medication and respected my choice. Grace is a wise and compassionate person, who knows the complex nature of the fragile psyche and the mystery and strength of the soul. She was precisely the source for healing I needed, and I humbly thank God every day for her.

She capably navigated me through the rocky channels of PTSD and the deep grief I felt over mother's death and the others. We tried to tackle the many problems I had with understanding Clay, but answers evaded us both. It would be some time before we learned what type of disorder was playing havoc with me and my life. Her gift of reassurance was invaluable in reclaiming my emotional equilibrium. Regardless of how absurd the stories of my experiences with Clay, she believed me. She never made me feel paranoid or unhinged when it came to Clay's actions. Grace's gentle counsel safeguarded my somewhat fragile emotional and spiritual well-being. I was in the company of an angel.

## CHAPTER 13

*"There was a child went forth every day, And the first object he look'd upon, that object he became."*
— *There Was a Child Went Forth*, Walt Whitman

I managed to survive my frightening round trip to the river Styx and was feeling stronger, but having trouble trying to forgive Clay for his callous treatment of me during my darkest hours. I saw him more as a detriment to a spiritual and emotionally healthy existence than a partner. I learned an important lesson about this marriage—Clay was never going to be part of any solution to any problem, he was the problem.

Never once did he come to me and say, "I am so sorry to have made you doubt yourself, and I am sorry that I wasn't there for you when you needed someone so desperately after your mother and friends died." Those words would have made his stock soar and he would have secured my heart forever. But it hasn't happened and I suspect it never will.

My children were on their own and, thank God, managing quite well without me. The people I had talked to, saw almost daily, were gone. The more I lost, the more there was of Clay.

I honestly didn't know how to live with this man. I spent many hours trying to come up with some solution to the question: how can I continue to live with someone who is apparently so incompatible with me and the style of life I desperately need to survive and be happy?

I told him I was tired of not being treated as a wife and tired of him not seeing me as desirable or saying affirmative and loving things to make me feel loved or desirable. Tell me I'm hot or sexy once in awhile. I was sick of being a celibate wife. I felt humiliated that I had to even tell him that for the thousandth time.

That summer we had a heat wave; temperatures were in the triple digits. A week after my rant about his neglect, Clay came home from work, put down his briefcase and stood in front of me. I thought he was ready to deliver a comment on the weather or the news when he blurted, "You look hot." "No, I turned the A/C down and I'm comfortable." He stood there stupefied for a moment and then went upstairs. It was a few minutes later before I realized what he was trying to do, but the moment was gone and would never come around again. That's the way it worked with him. He would bungle and I would forgive, I would bungle and I would never be granted a second chance.

I was a tourist in his world and he was a visitor to mine; our relationship felt tenuous and temporary. It seems now, I was always waiting for the marriage to begin, to take off and feel normal and real in place of surreal and hollow.

I spent the last twenty years walking on wall-to-wall carpet made entirely out of egg shells, and as with anything that requires that much restraint and care, it gets old and extremely exhausting.

Over the next couple of years (let's face it, he was all that was left), I tried to communicate with him about my needs and my vision for our marriage, but the same old invisible partition was there repelling me and defeating my sincere desire to bond with the unusual person I married.

During this time of reconciliation, I planned to make some intimate dinners and select some romantic movies (I actually believed if he saw how other men seduced and made love to women, he would get the hint), but even this was too subtle for him. The kids once sat our dog in front of the TV and tried to get him to watch a program about canines, thinking he would get excited about it—nope, exactly like Clay and the movies, he gave us a blank look and wandered back to his food bowl.

I was trying to make lemonade out of the lemons I had been handed. I felt that it was too late to reconstruct the marriage, but there was a chance to have a life I could survive. I was afraid to ask him for any more involvement; his answer, like others in the past, would be disappointing or devastating—two great choices. I also began to suspect from his behavior toward me, all Clay wanted or needed from me was my help to replicate his childhood home and play the role of "mom."

At this point, even I knew this was the perfect definition of insanity: doing the same thing over and over and expecting different results.

Two of the only remaining positives about Clay I felt were laudable and workable, he was still around and faithful, although he would stare at other women—all heterosexual men did that, right? Except Clay's facial expression showed no hint of pleasure; it was a frozen stare lacking any appreciation. An example of how misleading his stare could be from his intent was that distressed women friends would come to me and ask if he was mad at them. I would politely interrupt his obvious and embarrassing reverie on many social occasions so as not to alarm the object of his fantasy and steer him away to another conversation or introduction. I could always tell when he zeroed in on an unsuspecting female—he stood very still with intense concentration and a fixed expression; it reminded me of when my children were in diapers and had that look, which alerted me that they were about to poop.

Clay would never stare at me that way, but he would stalk me around the house and I would catch him snooping. He was the consummate spy. He wanted to know everything going on but didn't dare ask. It was his weird nature not to openly confront people; he would skulk around on the perimeter to cloak his interest. It must have occurred to him that he could ask questions to find out what he wanted to know—in most circumstances, people like to talk about themselves to an interested listener, but he never acted on it. He didn't ask personal questions, not even of me. Like a ghost spy, he preferred to remain clandestine while gathering his peculiar data. I think he believes asking questions is an embarrassing act of stupidity.

The only consolation was my belief he had never been unfaithful. But even this would be ripped from me in the most demoralizing way.

In order to put my time to good use, I learned how to use his computer and also found another source of frustration. I worked hard to understand how to use something whose internal machinations I couldn't see—like Clay. The damn thing didn't respond to normal requests—like Clay. And learning which program opened which file would drive me to tears and junk food. I learned to use the keyboard and navigate the internet.

Ah, yes, the internet. There I discovered why Clay was spending hundreds of hours over the years enthralled with it. I had been under the impression he was working on job related assignments and I, the considerate wife, tip-toed around the house so as not to disturb him. I didn't bother him to help me with any household chores, and most nights I ate by myself and went to bed alone, as usual, so he could excel at his career. I couldn't understand how someone could spend nine or ten hours at work and come home and then work many more hours on that soul-sucking piece of technology. He had in the past jumped up from the dinner table with guests present and run upstairs to his computer, never to resurface to say good-night to our friends. This had gone on for years, eight to be exact, ever since he stopped having sex with me.

One day, quite by accident, I stumbled on to the answer to all the above questions—internet porn. But it wasn't just porn, it was the nature of the porn—S&M and B&D. I was sickened by what I saw. I shouldn't have been shocked: I had suspected him of pedophilia years before and found his stash of magazines, books, and videos in the same vein, but they didn't rival this degree of human depravity. We had talked about it at the time, and I told him how this made me sick and it lowered my respect for him, and stupid me I thought that was the end of it when he threw it all in the trash. At least now I knew where all his sexual energy was focused.

For many years I believed him to be asexual and then I thought he was gay, and now I saw him as a pervert. I also remembered his smug and arrogant response to my question about how he could go for such long periods of time without making love, "You must be needier than me." Bastard! He had an outlet, and once more, the gullible one was being faithful to my vow of "forsaking all others." I didn't want to kill him myself, I wanted to throw him to a pack of starved wolves and then toss him into the worst part of hell. Lorena Bobbitt was looking like a holy woman—and the patron saint of scorned women.

We were back in the principal's office; he sat slumped in his chair and I sat across from him trying to dialogue with the egomaniacal and willful perpetrator of the most heinous crime against my female-centric heart.

"Clay, why would you do this when I told you how much it hurt me?" As usual, the contrite blob with bowed head uttered his only defensive response, "I'm sorry. I didn't know I was being unfaithful."

"How do you think it makes me feel to know that this is what I have to compete with for your affection?" I exploded.

"But I look at older women too."

I wanted to kick, no, stomp him in the crotch. "Clay, whether the other party is two or three dimensional, old or young, it takes you out of the marital bed and away from me, your wife. You've ignored me and my needs. How is that not being unfaithful?"

Then he attempted to compartmentalize his actions and excuse them.

"But, I love you," he whined. His attempt at this childish and flimsy reconciliation infuriated me.

"Well, you sure do have a weird way of showing it. You spent the entirety of our marriage gratifying yourself and left me alone in the bedroom, tearing myself apart trying to figure out what I did to make you reject me, and when I asked what was wrong, you lied. How exactly is that love?"

"I'm sorry."

"So, I must conclude from your statement, that love has nothing to do with sex and vice versa? And based on that reasoning, I should be able to have sex with anyone, real or virtual, as long as I love you, and it's okay with you?"

"Well, no. Not with someone …r…real," he hiccupped at me.

"So, it would have been fine with you from the beginning when you expected we were going to have a sex life, but I arbitrarily changed the rules and decided without informing you first, I was going to redirect my affection and sexual energy to another person, real or otherwise, and neglect you?"

"No." He was uncomfortable wearing my shoes but was still unable to empathize with the pain he was inflicting.

"I'm sorry."

"Yes, you are. And FYI, two dimensional won't do it for me; I need a real person." I stormed out of the room; shaking with a rage I never knew I had.

I wanted to take the vision of him at that minute, as well as every past frame with his face in it, and vomit it from my memory—forever.

This ordeal was as vivid and terrifying as if he had sliced me open with a cold steel blade and had reached in as far as possible with his cruel greedy hands and grabbed my viscera, slowly and deliberately ripping them out, and as I bled, presented me with my own bloody beating heart.

If he had at anytime been honest with me about his repulsive sexual proclivities, maybe we could have worked things out sans the S&M and B&D. Maybe. I believe if I can understand something, it stands a chance of being accepted. I asked him how he became hooked on these two aberrant sexual styles; his answer made some sense, but was still unacceptable. He said when he was young this was the only sexual information he had access to on his own. I concluded his love map had been vandalized early and this type of pornography was permanently imprinted on his brain. However, Clay had usurped the opportunity for amends through his selfish and furtive behavior, the damage was done. He resolved the problem by giving me my own computer. Idiot!

From then on I had to continuously wash my mind of all the sickening images I had of his addiction to the vulgar lust for the cruel debasement of other human beings.

Then another new image, unbidden and unsubstantiated popped up, it was of Clay as a child sitting at a table and methodically tearing the wings off live flies, helpless creatures for which he had complete and absolute power. I didn't like this person and I remembered his statement to the therapist about his feeling of being only thirteen years old. From then on, it was how I saw him and I knew that I would never be able to think of him as a sexual partner again, but only as a child who will never grow up or be capable of becoming a husband.

Anything else would be pedophilia.

CAROLYNN WOODS

## CHAPTER 14

*"What can't be cured must be endured."*

—My Grandma

It's always darkest before the dawn, or so the saying goes, and I had waited for twenty years for the sun to rise and illuminate the mystery which continued to vex me on a daily basis, namely, Clay.

In the spring of 2003, our local newspaper ran an article about a family in our community who had a son with autism. The story revealed how difficult life had become for the parents of this child who could express only two emotions: anger and frustration. I was more than familiar with these volatile expressions. They were the only emotions Clay showed—the only two!

This got me to thinking about Clay, but I couldn't connect the dots from autism to Clay. The article described a few of the same behaviors I saw in Clay, but along with enlightenment came confusion. Like many people, I had heard of autism, but believed it only affected young children. I never heard them described as anything other than tragically debilitated and read nothing further about them beyond their early childhood. I naturally assumed they were institutionalized and this is where my understanding of autism ended.

I am also aware there has been little effort to educate the general public beyond this narrow perspective. Most of what people hear today about autism only covers its statistical presence in our country: one child in every 144 children born each day will be diagnosed with autism. If this statistic were given for a highly virulent form of plague, convinced we were in the middle of an epidemic, we would all be running to health agencies and beating the doors down demanding treatment and preventative care. Autism should be considered at a pandemic level. It transcends race, nationality, and socio-economic strata. There are many theories as to the cause of autism, but they are complex and vary widely among researchers in the field of Spectrum Disorders.

I learned there are "degrees" of autism along a spectrum. On one end, there are those individuals who are visibly disabled—unable to communicate, make eye contact, incessantly rocking or flapping their hands, but at the far end of the spectrum are individuals, like Clay, who are considered "high functioning." At his level of ability, these people grow up, marry and carry their disorder into the nursery. This form of autism is referred to as a "hidden disorder," and this is why I and so many other women missed the signs of this devastating condition from our very first encounter with these men.

After reading the newspaper article, I felt I had my first solid lead to follow and a new direction for my search. I staggered home from local libraries at least once a week with stacks of books filled with information about autism—many contained only a short paragraph with the word "Autism," along with a short medical definition. I was speed reading and making notes, but felt highly disappointed by the texts, which exclusively described the clinical symptoms of children. I could find nothing addressing autism in adults; this void supported my notion that either the disorder or the afflicted individual disappeared in some manner (death or institutionalization) prior to reaching adulthood. Eventually I stumbled across the term "Asperger's Syndrome," and that was the key to the door that would unlock the mystery which had tormented me for a third of my life.

Newly equipped with a name for what I believed Clay had, I began a dedicated search for more information. I found some sparse anecdotal accounts from individuals and some clinical information on the internet, but nothing that answered my questions: Where do I go? Who do I talk to? Are there Autismologists?

I went to our local chapter of the Autism Society, trusting, at last, I would get the help I desperately needed. When I arrived at the office, no one looked up from their paperwork long enough to greet me. I looked around the room, which housed two desks, one occupied and one vacant, and a table in the center of the room presently being used by two people eating their lunch and reading. I waited several minutes hoping someone would approach and ask me if they could be of help. Impatient for assistance, I wandered down a hallway until I found a small office with an open door occupied by a slight woman in her mid-thirties and lightly tapped on the door. I cleared my throat to get her attention; she stopped shuffling through a pile of papers and looked surprised to see someone standing in her doorway. I introduced myself and told her what I needed: specifically, a support group and information about Asperger's Syndrome. "I have a son with autism and his father has it too. I divorced him because I got tired of doing it all and doing it alone." I think I commiserated with her over her predicament and waited for something else, I'm not certain what, but that wasn't it. "Do you have any information about adults with the disorder?" No longer looking at me but focusing her attention back to her pile of papers, she pointed back toward the room with the lunch table, "There is a bookcase in there, it has books you can buy." I found the narrow four-shelf bookcase and rummaged through the available pamphlets and books, finally finding one, "The Other Half of Asperger Syndrome" by Maxine Aston. That was the sum total of help I received from the Autism Society. Before leaving, I paid membership dues and insisted on leaving my name and phone number in the event a support group became available; I even offered to start one. I heard nothing for four years.

I hurried home, eager to read the book and hoping it would help me to understand why Clay was the way he was and prayed it would also show me how to proceed with a marriage that had long since ceased to be one. It didn't help with the marriage issue, but what it did give me was unexpected and invaluable: it gave me the validation I so deeply required to believe I wasn't hysterical or delusional about Clay or our bizarre relationship.

I found great comfort and renewed self-confidence just knowing I had not imagined or exaggerated my circumstances. I learned, too, I was not alone. There were many more just like Clay, which unfortunately meant there were many more women, like me, out there experiencing the very same self doubts and emotional pain.

During one of the darkest periods of my life, I was fortunate to have Grace Rowlson as my therapist, who gave me encouragement and helped me find my strength and determination to return to the land of the living—she was the dawn in my new life and Maxine Aston became the high noon. I was blessed to have found these two exceptional women. Ms. Rowlson was my spiritual and emotional support and Ms. Aston, an author and psychologist who practices in the U.K., whom I have never met, gave me the courage to write my story.

Although I had an answer as to what destroyed my relationship with Clay, which in itself was an immeasurable boost to my self confidence, I had one more devastatingly difficult fact to assimilate about autism: there is no cure.

## CHAPTER 15

*"Between my brain and me there is always a layer that I cannot penetrate."*

—Jules Renard

The term "incurable" did not register with me, not immediately or completely. It took a month or more for the full impart of that word to sink in. It took even longer for it to burrow down into the abstract domicile of inner turmoil where the mind and the heart negotiate for resolution. I felt relieved of a monstrous burden; I had a name for Clay's condition. Finally, something concrete I could understand; the adversary was in the open and not hidden in shadows where it would ambush and taunt me—invisible and menacing. I didn't feel happy about Clay's diagnosis—he wasn't going to get better and I feared neither would I. It didn't magically erase all the devastating memories, heal gaping wounds or shrink scars. He had hurt me deeply and I wasn't confident I could overcome the emotional damage he and his disorder had caused.

Knowing the truth didn't fix anything. I felt he was responsible for his actions, and I continue to feel this way. If this had been any other disease or handicap, he would have my complete sympathy, understanding and support. With this particular disorder when the person is physically and mentally functional but arrogantly basks in his own self-proclaimed superiority, the psyche's perception remains one of betrayal. I willingly admit his disorder wasn't his fault. Regardless of how I struggled to put this information into a compassionate and practical light, I continued to feel I had been duped. You don't get over Asperger's, whichever side you reside on.

Only on rare occasions were Clay and I able to talk about the diagnosis, and he surprised me by saying, "At least I know it isn't my fault." I was curious about what he meant; naturally, he added no further insight. Had he always felt there was something wrong with him and suddenly felt vindicated? I don't know, I can only presume. Clay has never tried to tell his side of the story and this left only me to investigate on my own, spending years in the attempt to define and understand him. I looked at him, seeing a child with a bowed head; he looked deflated and for the very first time I felt pity for him. I couldn't bring myself to say, "It's okay, we'll get through this," because I didn't know how to get through any of it. I was left hanging with many more but quite different questions about this disorder. I thought since he knew he was responsible for most of the misunderstandings between us and for his disruptive and hurtful behavior, I wanted to believe he would use this new self-awareness as an agent for change.

For a time, we danced our familiar routine of the non-musical version of "Approach and Avoidance." He temporarily dressed in sackcloth, while I took the attitude of wait and see. I eagerly placed the onus on him; I had carried it long enough. There were minute changes; one was trying to control his temper and the other, communication. He quickly became disenchanted with the amount of effort it took and would have a meltdown, leaving me to walk on eggshells. He had all the charm and grace of a leopard walking a tightrope while simultaneously trying to change his spots.

The few times when he was willing and I wasn't seething with my own anguish, provoked either by him or the disorder, which had robbed me of a husband, we were able to sit down and talk about Asperger's. I knew he was being honest when he said, "I know I can't say the things you need to hear, I feel them, but there's this glass wall I can't get through." At that moment, I felt my heart relax and accepted his sincere confession of complete helplessness—the first he ever offered. I wish his statement could have healed our pained history, but it soon evaporated in the heat of his next rage.

I would look at Clay and easily compare him to my son and grandsons in early adolescence. It was a startling and accurate template. To me he was thirteen years old and would always remain so.

They were all clumsy, unkempt, with voracious appetites and an insatiable need to sleep. If I dared to interrupt their routine and to ask for help with a chore, they were disagreeable and churlish and vocal. They could also be surprisingly pleasant and eager to help if the mood struck; it was difficult to predict which response would be forthcoming. They lacked the inclination to offer help. They would have to be asked repeatedly to walk the dogs, take out the trash, or clean their room. They were not self-motivated to do anything for anyone. They had a furtive and heightened interest in sex but no clue as to how to go about seducing the opposite sex, combined with a heart stopping fear of any possible encounter to that end. They kept their distance from females but gawked whenever the opportunity presented itself. They had a devout interest in all the current game technology: x-boxes, Wii, interactive computer games and fantasy literature. They talked exclusively and excessively about these topics. They would save their Christmas and birthday money for new videos games with the fevered anticipation of an addict about to score street drugs.

They hugged me if I asked for it, and when I insisted, would grudgingly sit and have impatient conversations when they would rather be in front of a screen of some description—they lacked a huge chunk of the social graces. This is where the resemblance to Clay ended. None of my grandchildren have Asperger's, but at this stage of development they had a lot more in common with Clay than I did. Along with disgustingly typical adolescent male behavior was the sheer joy of watching these "free range" boys cut up, have belching contests and affectionately tease me. They were not above breaking the rules, not the serious ones anyway, but they would push the envelope. They tested their parent's authority and patience, but never stepped over the line into disrespect. Boys—normal, healthy kids—you gotta love them.

The symptoms of Asperger's Syndrome (I will use "AS" as an abbreviation), the very same which Clay exhibits and pushed me to the very edge of reality, are: inability to read non-verbal cues—difficulty interpreting and using body language, lacks executive and planning abilities, inappropriate social approaches and responses, lacks theory of mind (doesn't think that someone else thinks and fails to consider other's viewpoint), inability to make eye contact, inability to recognize the emotions, feelings and facial expressions of others, takes language literally—can't process sarcasm or metaphors, and shows limited ability in conversing. They also have trouble making friends. Most terrifying to me is they can't tell if you are in trouble and need help—forget the Heimlich maneuver if you are choking or need CPR during cardiac arrest; don't even count on a 911 call on your behalf unless you can tell them what to do. Add idiosyncratic special interests and difficulty managing negative feelings, especially anxiety, anger and depression, to the fact that they also lack empathy and are egocentric and voilá—you have Clay. If he had come with a full disclosure statement, a user's manual, or some other caveat, I would have never signed on for this bizarre journey into his alternative universe, and I don't believe any other woman would either.

## CHAPTER 16

*"...Trust the instinct to the end, though you can render no reason."*

—Ralph Waldo Emerson

When Clay told me about the "glass wall" in his head that wouldn't allow him to express his feelings, I knew he wasn't aware he was telling me something important. I didn't understand why at the time, but his statement niggled at my brain for months; it kept chirping in my head with the same relentless demand as a smoke alarm with a weak battery.

In the past, he demonstrated frustration over his inability to respond appropriately when I would try to present my case for an intimate relationship and my desire to hear the words which supported these emotions. He showed signs of severe physical distress—furiously rubbing his forehead, straining and struggling to find the words he couldn't speak. It was unnerving to watch a grown man grappling with something that should have come so easily in a relationship. It left me feeling like some kind of monster; expecting him to speak of loving feelings, while watching him writhe in pain at what I thought was a simple request not unheard of between two people. Instead of pursuing this encounter, which over time I realized was futile, and out of deference to his discomfort, I would leave the room feeling depressed and cheated.

Sometime later, as luck would have it, I was flipping through TV channels and caught a documentary about Kim Peek, the real life "Rain Man" from the movie with Tom Cruise and Dustin Hoffman. I was completely enthralled with the story of this unique human being. There were significant differences between Mr. Peek and Clay, like Peek's visible disabilities, but it was the similarities that caught and held my attention and curiosity.

Kim Peek, a man in his fifties, is described as a confounding mixture of disability and brilliance; in the world of neuroscience he is considered a "mega savant." Most savants have one dominating interest; Kim Peek has a vast appetite for knowledge and soaks up everything in his range of interests (a feature I saw in Clay and coined "Data dosing"). He can recall thousands of zip codes, area codes, dates, and innumerable facts and figures.

During one scene of the documentary, I watched as he demonstrated his amazing memory in the lecture hall of a university campus; students would ask him, "What day of the week was it on October 27th, 1582?" Without hesitation, "It was a Tuesday." And so it went until the audience ran out of questions and steam.

Naturally, neurologists are curious as to how the brain of this incredible individual works. Who wouldn't be? In 2005, several scientists from different disciplines worked together in overlapping investigations to produce a profile of Peek's mental makeup. A psychologist, Dr. Rita Jeremy, gave him a standardized I.Q. test and found he had trouble with tasks that require new thinking or where he can't recall facts from memory. The erratic results were inconclusive and Dr. Jeremy decided standardized tests cannot be applied to his unusual mentality.

Dr. Elliott Sherr, a neurologist, went over Peek's background and discovered he learned to read by the age of two, and although his was not a formal neurological assessment, he determined that Peek had difficulty following directions.

A neurological evaluation followed with the use of Diffusion Tensor Imaging; a recent tool added to the arsenal of diagnostic equipment to map brain functions. This procedure was administered by Neuroradiologist Dr. Pratik Mukherjee. The test revealed the two halves, or hemispheres, of Peek's brain weren't joined in the normal way; a condition known as ACC (Agenesis of the Corpus Callosum)—he was born without one.

Some people, like Peek, are missing the corpus callosum at birth (agenesis) and others are born with a partial or diminished corpus. There are also those who have had it surgically removed for medical reasons.

The corpus callosum is a bridge made up of fibers, approximately 200 million, connecting the left and right hemispheres of the brain and allows communication between these two giant processors, much like a network connection running different programs from the same input.

The left side of the body is wired to the right side of the brain and visa-versa; nature created this cross-over for whatever reason and it applies to vision, but not hearing.

In the 1970's, Roger Sperry, a Nobel Prize Laureate and psychobiologist from CalTech, conducted "split-brain" experiments, and the results of those studies are used to explain how Kim Peek was still able to function, at least in some areas, without his corpus.

Sperry's experiments involved the testing of a patient who, suffering from uncontrolled seizures, had an area of his brain surgically removed: the area was the corpus collosum, which was suspected of having developed lesions (short circuits) from intractable epilepsy. Today, new methods and technology make it possible to remove only a tiny portion of the corpus callosum from these patients.

Although the communications link between the two halves was severed, the patient's left and right brain hemispheres were functioning independently.

A series of tests were conducted: different visual and tactile information could then be presented to the patient's right or left side without the other side knowing. The results were astounding.

The right hand and eye utilizing the left brain could name an object, such as a pen, but the patient couldn't explain its purpose. Then it was shown to the left hand and eye utilizing the right brain, and the patient could explain and demonstrate its use. Further "split-brain" studies involving patients who had the corpus severed showed various functions of thought are physically separated and localized to a specific area on either the left or right side of the human brain. Sperry was able to show a conscious mind exists in each hemisphere.

He and his group showed by ingenious tests definite behavioral phenomena can be demonstrated following the split brain surgery. This work in "split brain" experiments continues and new discoveries are frequently published.

Upon completion of this "map" of the brain it became clear that each hemisphere had a characteristic way that it both interpreted the world and reacted to it.

The left brain is dominant in all functions involving the following: logic, attention to detail, facts, speech (words and language), present and past, math and science, comprehension, acknowledging order and patterns, perception, knowing the names of objects, but not their functions, reality awareness, forms strategies, practical and safe behaviors.

The right brain, although mute, contributes emotional context to language and is only capable of simple addition (up to 20), but is superior to the left hemisphere in the following: feelings, is holistic or "big picture oriented, it's where imagination rules, it sees symbols and images, is aware of present and future, comprehends philosophy and religion, can "get it"—jokes and sarcasm (i.e., meaning), believes, appreciates, spatial perception (understanding maps), knows an object's function, recognizes faces, is fantasy based, can present possibilities, understands the abstract, uses empathy, impetuous and risk taking behaviors.

Until the discovery of the duality of consciousness by Sperry, it was considered doubtful whether the right brain was even conscious. By devising methods of communicating with the right brain, Sperry could show that "it is indeed a conscious system in its own right; perceiving, thinking, remembering, reasoning, willing and emoting, all at a characteristically human level, and ... both the left and the right hemisphere may be conscious simultaneously in different, even in mutually conflicting, mental experiences that run along a parallel." Each hemisphere is still able to learn after being severed, but each has no access to what the other side has learned or experienced.

Successful attempts at reconnecting these neural fibers in animals with a severed corpus showed the previous behavior and responses were "hardwired" into the brain from birth and would always remain so.

It was amazing to watch Peek and also sad to realize regardless of his incredible and unmatched mental calisthenics, he had no "real world" talents or abilities. I could see many of Kim Peek's traits in Clay, the Google-like brain and the inept social ability: the childlike quality, the awkward posture, and stilted language. When Peek was introduced to the faculty members of the campus where he was a guest, he shook hands and said, "You are a great man" or "great lady," whichever the case, using the same scripted language I was accustomed to hearing from Clay as in "You look hot" or "You look pretty."

Kim's father, a parent possessing great courage, selflessness, and patience, elected not to institutionalize his young son after Kim's mother abandoned him, but instead became his lifelong caretaker. He dresses him, cooks for him and cares for him in similar ways one would a child of five or six years of age. Kim claims that he and his father have the same shadow. His father is in his eighties and I am certain he worries about his son's future in a world without him—the same concerns I hear and read about from the parents of children with autism.

Since autism and AS are neurological disorders, it seemed a natural progression for me to investigate the brain, or specifically the corpus, as a possible source for the disorder Clay and I were struggling with on a daily and visceral basis. The brain held a tremendous attraction for me since it evidently was the only organ in our marriage in "play."

I couldn't help but feel there was a strong connection between Clay's condition and the state of his corpus callosum. I also learned that the symptoms of ACC are typically identical to those for Asperger's: motor, language, or cognitive delays, poor motor coordination, sensitivity to tactile sensations, and social challenges. They lack insight into one's own behavior, lack awareness of others' feelings, misunderstanding social cues, limited sophistication of humor, and difficulty imagining consequences of behavior. ACC requires the same team of professionals and support agencies as autism.

During my years with Clay, I always sensed a disconnection. I would jokingly say to him, "I'm sending you back to your mother. You're not done, yet." At the time I didn't understand where that came from or why it felt true. I understand now that

I had a perception of him as an adult, but I always felt the presence of an underdeveloped and elusive entity. We didn't interact in the manner two adults in love did, we intersected at sharply odd angles. He constantly put me off by withholding (I thought deliberately) the emotional responses I needed and expected in a loving mate. Even a small child can express feelings of fear, pain, joy, empathy and love; qualities Clay seemed to have no access to and failed to reciprocate. I remember the frustration I felt when the most elementary encounters required so much energy and explanation to get through when it should have been easily and universally understood between mature adults.

I could see a physically grown man and would gravitate toward him expecting adult behavior: sex, comfort, conflict resolution, sharing of ideas, goals, dreams, and spirituality, but I would hit the proverbial brick (or perhaps, I should say, "glass") wall.

I sensed there was some level on which he was trying to process the emotions and thoughts I was lobbing at him, but there was a hesitation, a delay followed by his fits of anger or frustration. He drifted away convinced I was not capable of understanding him, and he was correct—I didn't, but it wasn't his intellect or his esoteric subject matter, it was his behavior, attitude and lack of "humanity", I was searching for and couldn't locate.

I always sensed the presence of "another" in our marriage. At first I suspected it was another woman, but with my new insight into the corpus, I realized with the same intense jolt as a crack of thunder, it wasn't a presence, it was a—void.

I began constructing new theories about AS and Clay; I could for the first time logically and clearly see where our differences lay—in our brain pans.

Had I met Clay when we were both in early adolescence, he would have appeared quite normal to me. All girls my age knew all boys at that age were "goofy." They were socially inept, physically awkward, and vested in their own world of special interests and painfully shy, but also curious about the opposite sex. Sex was out of the equation, so it wasn't a problem, then. Then somewhere around this time of maturation and development, I and my sisters sprinted ahead, leaving boys in a haze of evolutionary dust, so to speak, and boys like Clay even further behind in a blinding fog of delayed maturation.

He physically and intellectually matured but remained emotionally stunted while his brethren learned through risky behavior and a process of trial and error the "tricks of the trade" for the seduction of females. Clay, left without peers or older brothers, was on his own to decipher the nuances of male-female relationships. The only access he had to sexual instruction was "girly magazines" and adult book stores. This questionable but popular method of sex education taught Clay the mechanical and physical aspects of the act, but didn't teach him the most crucial lessons about male-female relationships.

During courtship and mating, other men were learning they had to recognize the functions of their partner's right brain (I'm certain they weren't thinking in those terms) to navigate and utilize it to gain entry into the female mystique to be rewarded with her sexual favors and/or her hand in marriage. Although most men will tell you in a New York minute, "You're the sexiest woman in the world," or "Let me take you to a chick flick, baby"— these sexually deferred detours are not their favorite route to the desired destination; however, it is the safest and the surest.

Modern man has learned his lessons about the evolved fairer sex well—you've gotta romance the brain—always start at the top, guys. The brain is the ultimate sex organ, all the other stuff is merely accessible peripheral equipment.

Sometime during Clay's development (around 12 or 13), for whatever reason—bio-chemically or genetically, his brain began to function predominately and, it appears, almost exclusively, in his left hemisphere, while his right hemisphere simply became ballast.

Whether this mysterious catalyst was triggered from the exposure to the modeling examples displayed and encouraged by his left hemispheric parents, or was an unfortunate combination of all these things programmed into his DNA to cease development of the corpus and thus ceased to nourish his right brain at adolescence, I don't know.

What I do know is how Clay interacted with me. The "glass" wall became an impediment to his ability to express his feelings and other right brain functions and stands as an unrelenting sentinel posted between the two worlds where most of us easily and constantly transmit and receive messages, which allow us to communicate in multiple and emotionally satisfying ways.

I didn't see this impediment as a glass wall but rather a chasm, too wide for him to leap across, leaving him stranded on a small isolated island and missing a huge chunk of what rocks the world for the rest of us. I can understand the frustration of feeling loving, caring and nurturing emotions and the need to convey them to another but being unable to utter the words. In Clay's situation, if the message carrying this emotion can't find a network connection, like an email, it would languish in the outbox, never sent and therefore never received.

Learning more about the hemispheric realms of the brain made me reconsider the question of Clay's atheism. He had little if any access to the emotional or spiritual. Is the right brain the conduit for God and the many philosophies and theologies regarding life, afterlife, faith and spirituality?

What can a person who is dependent upon those spoken and demonstrated emotions do when they never come? This was part of my ongoing conundrum with Clay; I would have to always give him the benefit of the doubt and assume his feelings and actions were coming from a spiritual and caring place, even when he was raging, arrogantly blustering, ignoring, and neglecting me, which action am I to believe? Even those who are deaf or mute can use sign language to replace the spoken word, but when someone has no verbal or tactile means of communicating their feelings and this person is your spouse, life becomes empty and inconsolable.

This is why I feel lonely and cheated. We seem to represent two different species unable to communicate in the way that matters most in a marriage. In his role as husband he is as unsuited for me as if he were an aardvark.

## CHAPTER 17

*"...The child is father to the man."*
                                —William Wordsworth

I wish Clay could have had an fMRI (functional Magnetic Resonance Imaging) to solve to my question about his brain structure and function, but I knew there was no practical reason to pursue it for two reasons: cost, and it wouldn't change anything. Clay is "hardwired" into his left brain and will always remain so. MRIs are expensive and no HMO is going to approve a procedure simply to satisfy my theory. I have since discovered some research which recently surfaced and may support my theory.

Two studies and the resulting theory were the work of Marcel Just, Ph.D., D.O., Professor of psychology at Carnegie Mellon University, Pittsburgh, Pennsylvania, and Ellen Minshaw, MD., Professor of Psychiatry and Neurology at the University of Pittsburgh, School of Medicine, and their colleagues. The study showed that autism may involve a lack of normal sized connections (the corpus callosum) and coordination in separate areas of the brain.

Other research by neurological scientists has shown the brains of autistics are significantly smaller or larger in some regions compared to normal brains.

We were fortunate to get a simple diagnosis of AS for Clay. The guideline for diagnostic services is reserved almost exclusively for children from three years old through twenty-two years of age. Most professionals in the field don't bother with older individuals with AS because they are considered very highly functional and assume they fare well enough in society—although, I beg to differ, they require either spousal, parental or agency support

The agencies that provide these services use their financial and human resources to test, diagnose, treat and support the families of children with CA (classical autism) throughout the spectrum to HFA (high functioning autism) and AS (Asperger's Syndrome) in a restricted age range. During the process of having a child diagnosed, it is usually revealed that one or both parents are on the spectrum.

The observations made in 1944 in Vienna, Austria by Dr. Hans Asperger, a pediatrician, were the result of his classifying children, mostly boys, under his care as "autistic"—from the Greek word auto, meaning self. His observations also included the parents of these children who shared the same traits.

Families going in the door may come out with more than they bargained for in the search for answers. The mother, or in some cases the father, knows that she has been the primary parent and has struggled with a spouse who lacks independent parenting skills or is idling away in front of a computer while she runs a three ring circus in the home and can't imagine why she is always exhausted, alone and on the verge of falling apart. Unlike the non-breeding wives in Asperger's marriages (like me), she will have an army of professionals for support, education and mentoring to assist her and her children in her ongoing lifelong battle with this disastrous disorder. The Octomom is an example of the huge need for outside support. She has three children on the spectrum and how many of her octuplets will require these services is still unknown.

If I had had a child with Clay, I would have been aware much sooner of the core problems in our marriage—a steep price to pay for insight. Fortunately, I convinced him to have a vasectomy right after we were married. I truly believe I would have run screaming for the hills if I had Clay, Melinda, and another affected child to raise in addition to my three children. In fact, I know I would; eventually we did have another one on the spectrum.

Clay's daughter Melinda married; she and her husband remained childless for a decade. Years earlier, Melinda dropped out of college because she thought she knew more than the institution could offer but required many tutors and she kept getting lost on campus. After she married, she worked full time as a waitress and raised and trained her seven dogs (her special interest).

She had one miscarriage and around the time she was pregnant again, we learned of Clay's disorder and that it was genetic and probably hereditary. Of course I had long ago suspected this was the case as I frequently descended down the Rabbit hole.

Melinda had a high-risk pregnancy but did quite well. Her husband, a part time musician, worked in his family business and when they opened a new office in the western part of our state, Rick was relocated and went ahead to set up the business and left Melinda behind to sell their house. She was late into her last trimester and they still had not found a rental property that would accept seven dogs.

She already transferred her medical records to a new ob-gyn over three hundred miles away, but refused to get rid of three or four of her dogs. Rick was working, house hunting, and driving back and forth weekly trying to sell their property. Melinda stubbornly refused to help facilitate the transfer by adopting out her animals and was looking at a rapidly approaching delivery date.

She stubbornly maintained her desires over anything or anyone else's best interest. I felt sorry for Rick; he was shouldering a huge responsibility with little help. Finally, three weeks before she was delivered by cesarean she relented and gave up three dogs.

She and Rick had a beautiful boy they named Steven. Shortly after he was born, we chose to tell Melinda about Clay's disorder and that it was hereditary. We suggested she tell her pediatrician so that he could monitor the baby's progress and development. I also wanted to persuade her to get a diagnosis for herself, but realized it would only alienate her. After all, I was dealing with a very superior family who didn't admit to any imperfections. In fact, in this clan I was the "special needs" person.

I often thought of myself as the character, Cousin Marilyn (not for any physical resemblance) in the "Munsters," the 1960's

TV comedy series with the family whose characters were an ensemble of all the monsters who appeared in horror movies from the 1940s and '50s. There was Herman, the husband, his wife Lily, grandpa Dracula, and their son, a young vampire. A pet dragon lived under the staircase. They were a macabre but functional family in the most bizarre ways. Marilyn was the only "normal" looking and behaving relative in the bunch, but she constantly bemoaned her inability to fit in with her eccentric, offbeat family. Unfortunately, I could relate.

We also informed Ellen, Clay's mother, who immediately began disclaimers for her side of the genetic contribution. When Clay told her he had hypertension, "It didn't come from my side of the family." Then when he told her about his rectal polyps, "We never had anything like that in my family," and on she went. All her family was deceased and beyond scrutiny, but I had my suspicions. She wasn't taking the rap for anything except the superlative qualities she felt she possessed; anything else was someone else's fault.

I was deeply concerned for this new baby. Melinda never showed any interest or patience with younger children, and as far as I knew, she hadn't babysat and had never changed a diaper. When she was around infants she kept her distance and never offered to hold or cradle a baby like most women are eager to do. She often spoke with disdain about children in general.

I knew that she was quite dependent upon Rick to raise this child. As with her past "hobbies," the family would have to support her and carry the financial burden of her self-centric interests. She and the newborn went to his office everyday and when they all went home, Rick did the cooking. She didn't clean house—she wasn't a homemaker, she was a thirty-three year old child playing with dolls. When I asked her what she did now that she had a baby, she couldn't answer except to say, "Rick has to help, too."

I knew from my past history with her, that Rick would be the primary parent and his parents, who lived nearby, would have to take on the duty of constant support for Melinda. Rick's parents had already lost one grandchild to severe mental retardation and had another on the spectrum.

I was happy to see that she was breast feeding, but dismayed to learn that when Melinda decided to go "green" by using cloth diapers (good for her), she didn't rinse them out, but would throw the soiled diapers in the washer with the dried stool still in them. I was hesitant to cuddle or diaper the baby—not knowing what bacteria was lurking in his clothing gave me pause. But as the saying goes, "God looks after drunks and little children," and this little guy seemed to be pretty healthy.

She tried to be a good mother and read books about parenting. She taught Steven baby sign language when he was around one year old, which restricted verbal interaction for the rest of us and excluded us from having him alone. Melinda had to stay present to interpret for us and breast feed. We couldn't feed him and he couldn't communicate with us.

What concerned me the most about her unconventional parenting skills was what appeared to me to be a total lack of intuition and nurture. I saw what bore a strong resemblance to the same methods she used to "train" her dogs. She micromanaged little Steven every minute he was awake. I wanted to tell her, "Leave him alone and let him be a child." She was constantly commanding either Steven or the dogs, it was hard to tell which she was giving these directives to, "Sit," "Eat," "Stay" or "Come here." Once I heard her tell little Steven when he reached up his arms for an embrace, "No, you've had your hug for today." I wanted to cry for this child.

Steven responded to me and I to him, he was an adorable child. I would hold out my arms and he would sail into them smiling from ear to ear. I can't resist children and have to talk to them wherever or whenever I see one; in a restaurant, in a store or out walking.

Once during a visit with Melinda and the boys, we were watching "Happy Feet" with Steven when he asked why penguins walked funny. I, trying to keep the answer simple so we could sit down and eat dinner, said, "Because that's the way God made them." Melinda shot me a look and contradicted my statement by saying, "No, Steven, that's the way they were made." I had momentarily forgotten referring to God is prohibited in front of the children.

I got the feeling Melinda, who now has a second son, used her children for an experimental project or hobby. She approaches motherhood as a job and not necessarily as a calling. When they visit, she immediately begins putting her boys through their paces like they were at a training trial for dogs. Steven, who is now five, has become a little professor like his grandfather Clay. When he plays with building blocks he lines them up in a straight line, demonstrating to me his lack of imagination. He requires a lot of energy and supervision from adults; we are constantly answering questions and making suggestions about what he can do next. There is never any "down" time with this child—it's exhausting. His curiosity and energy could easily be spent by playing with other children his age, but regrettably he doesn't have that privilege or opportunity. Melinda keeps him close to home and her, almost as if she is fearful of sharing him or allowing him to venture far from her control. I also see the simmering little demon of anger and frustration in his face and eyes when he doesn't get his way.

Melinda signed Steven up for soccer when he was four, but the poor child spent his entire time on the field running up and hugging the other players, so she withdrew him from the team.

Melinda is determined she is going to "home school" Steven. My heart crashed when she told me this. I hoped he would attend a traditional school where he would be exposed to other children and develop social skills and if required, evaluated for special educational needs. She's adamant about home schooling and is currently teaching him Latin for two or three hours a day. She never took Latin and rarely uses correct English grammar. I fear there is another little "Clay" in the making, and I know what his life will become and the life of his future love interest.

## CHAPTER 18

*"Allow me to furnish the interior of my head as I please, and I shall put up with a hat like everybody else's."*
—Henri Bergson

Ellen and Melinda are not the only women I know with Asperger's traits. My Goddaughter is also on the spectrum, as is her son. It took years for me to understand why she was so odd. When she lost her husband to melanoma when he was thirty-two, her in-laws took over the care and rearing of her son. She had difficulty parenting alone. She moved to Hawaii by herself and only sees her family every three or four years.

After twenty-six years in an Asperger's "living laboratory," I have developed a sixth sense about these individuals and can feel an atmospheric change when I am in their presence. There are many women on the spectrum, but they tend to fly under the radar and are a tiny bit more difficult to detect.

They are as deceptively camouflaged as the men on the spectrum, perhaps more so, since they possess somewhat better verbal and social skills. Asperger women, like AS men, can be extroverted or introverted; they can enjoy social interactions and on the surface appear passive and accommodating. These are not "take charge" type women; they require help and support with executive and planning functions like AS men. They can be easily led into situations that may be injurious to them. Trust is important to all people with AS; they can't comprehend the intentions of strangers and are reliant upon a loyal and trusted mentor to interpret these motives and actions. Normal men find these female AS traits attractive: a passive woman who will depend on them for protection and everything else and is accommodating, who thinks he is the ultimate, and will share male interests. Men also like the idea of a woman who requires no emotional preamble in the bedroom.

Women on the spectrum are as left brained as men. They prefer male company over females; I think they feel scrutinized and judged by other women—and they are because they are so different. Their conversational tone is similar to males—unemotional and fact driven. That is not to say that they are without emotions; they can have crying jags and fits when frustrated or angry like any other woman. The first thing I notice is they get nervous and giddy with new people even in a social setting. If they are professionals (teachers, professors, nurses, psychologists, physicians, computer engineers, dentists, etc.), they tend to take on a professional persona and have little to offer in the way of personal female relationships.

These gals are all business and don't appear comfortable outside of impersonal discussions. If the conversation does segue into intimate territory, they become evasive because they can't fathom the intent of women wanting to have deeply personal conversations—any personal exchange carries the danger of blowing their cover. If you make the cut, expect a long vetting process before you are trusted and considered a "safe" confidant.

I have been in several of these relationships and realize that they, too, like their male counterparts, can have a "helpless" quality, which can draw you in and before you can say, "Asperger" you're doing their chores because they are so overwhelmed or pitching in at the office and the next thing you know you've adopted a new puppy. At some point in any relationship when the "give and take" exchange arises, and with any friendship between women there is the expectation a friend is going have your back and be there for you as you have been for her, but soon enough it will become apparent that this a one-sided exercise; it's as though they are oblivious to your problems and need for support and empathy. They may offer, but when it comes down to it, they're outta there.

I have personally known more AS women than AS men, and I wouldn't at all be surprised to hear someday they compete statistically with men on the spectrum.

I had a friend who lost three husbands; she stayed in constant conflict with her adult children and depended on her friends for support, but offered none in return. Her first husband divorced her and her second died of a heart attack. She told me husband number two looked "gray" for three days. She obviously ignored his condition and was honestly shocked when he succumbed to a "sudden death." Husband number three died of a stroke while in the same room with her. He had been unable to have intercourse for some time, so she shuttled him off several months before to a doctor who recommended mega doses of vitamin E for a penile condition. Again, she was either unaware of what was happening or missed the signs of stroke, and there went husband number three.

After his death, she was very angry with everyone. I believe she didn't like not having a husband who would act as a buffer between her and the people she regularly offended and started arguments with over her demands. I witnessed this often. He was her protector who would take the flack and settle conflicts. My other friends saw her as selfish and self-centered, with little regard for the well being and feelings of others.

The reason I mention this is because people with AS can miss the signals and clues in situations that may be life-threatening to their children or spouses. Not that I believe they are intentionally neglectful, but they can't see and interpret some common danger signs the rest of us do.

A couple of years ago she told me that her youngest daughter's son was diagnosed with autism. It seems the people I have suspected as being on the spectrum pop up with the news of a child or grandchild being diagnosed with the disorder—hmmm.

The women as well as the men on the spectrum are devout believers in the "Rules," like Clay. After years of living with AS family members, I was able to understand the value and purpose of these rules and what exactly they meant to people with Asperger's, as opposed to what they mean to the majority of society.

The rules are essential guidelines used to govern their existence in the world. Because these individuals are unable to make decisions based on personal judgment or common sense which we employ every day and for every occasion requiring some decisive or executive action, they must use a default of constrained, non-arbitrary standards to navigate in the world of nonverbal cues and abstracts. The rules also serve the additional purpose of giving the AS individual the reassurance that when everyone observes these universal rules, they, too, can function equally well and feel confidently in step with everyone else. The rules about sharing are particularly favorable; if cookies are being passed around, you have to give everyone one. They will get their fair share and be treated like equals if everyone abides by the rules. It sounds childish, but that's the nature of AS. If anyone thinks the rules aren't important, just try breaking one. You will be in for the fight of your life with people who feel ultra-entitled. It also seems that once these particular rules are in place, they are forever imprinted onto the AS brain and will remain there forever, never re-evaluated for relevance in adult life or extenuating circumstances. I think the AS personality was the source for the phrase, "engraved in stone."

I have not found any chat rooms or websites for male spouses of AS women and often wonder what stories they would tell.

I have only a mild acquaintance with the neighbors across the street from me. The son is HFA and the mother, an elementary music teacher, I suspect has AS. I don't know the father very well, but have heard him make a couple of sarcastic and belittling remarks to his wife. After they moved into their new house, I spotted her on that miserably cold, rainy day from my window coming outside in the rain. Their garage door was open and she kept coming out carrying armfuls of packing paper, out through the garage, through the downpour, walking the length of the garage to the trash can at the back. The trash can is on wheels so I would have wheeled it into the garage and stayed out of the rain, but that's just what I'd do. She traipsed in and out all day sopping wet like a drowned cat. I just watched and shook my head and thought, how odd.

## CHAPTER 19

*"We think caged birds sing, when indeed they cry."*
—John Webster

There are many other women, their number may be in the millions, worldwide, caught up in this disorder—the spouses of AS men. The Autism community affectionately refers to people with AS as "Aspies," giving the impression of non-threatening, cuddly creatures; they are far from cuddly and far from non-threatening.

Aspies and those working in the field of autism like to refer to normal people in the clinically cold term, "NT's", for neurologically typical—so much for a love match.

I am not going to give up using the term "normal" for the majority of us, as, I feel, it conveys more than just a neurological inference.

Over two years ago I was able to join a support group with other spouses of Asperger's, and for those who were out of state, we offered telephone support; nothing replaces the comforting sound of a human voice. We began with a website and over time began cautiously meeting in person. We knew we were an underground demographic and our reluctance to become "known," coupled with our shame and the fear of discovery by our husbands made us a timid group, initially. It took a few meetings before we all felt safe and comfortable with our new "sisters" and opened up and began to speak frankly and honestly about our painful and disappointing marriages.

The first thing that always occurs when we meet a new member and tell her, "We understand and know what you've been through," is a cascade of tears while we wait patiently for her to release the deluge of emotions and the closeted feelings she's been harboring for years, and for some, decades. We wait patiently, too, for her to feel the love and acceptance she hasn't received from her spouse or anyone else for what seems an eternity.

Then we to try to work through the many destructive self-recriminations: why didn't I notice this disorder, why did I fall in love with him, why did I marry him, what's wrong with me, why didn't I leave, and why did I waste my life on this man who gives nothing back? We comfort each other with the indisputable truth—we were deluded by an invisible assailant. We didn't know any more about what awaited us in the beginning of our relationships than the people who bought passage on the Titanic.

Each of us struggled and suffered for years before finding out the truth about the "men" we married or discovered a forum where we can safely voice our concerns and ask each other questions. We, all, have gone the therapy route only to find there are no definitive answers or therapies for making these marriages work, only individual help for the normal spouse to learn how to rebuild a life for herself. We often left these conventional marital sessions with lower self-esteem—feeling less worthy and more alone. The support that is most beneficial is of the shared, human experience variety where one heart recognizes another's pain. It doesn't come from a textbook used by most professionals; it has to be applied with gentle recognition of specific wounds. It is often described as treading water for eons and then someone shows up with not only a life preserver, but a warm blanket and hot cocoa. It's beyond words. It's the first life affirming moment these women have experienced since they married their aardvarks.

Conventional therapists are very helpful in reconstructing the psyche to a realization of self and wholeness. I was lucky, I had Grace.

Some women want to stay in their marriage for various personal reasons: to get their career or finances in better shape, or their children are soon to be emancipated, and others want to become strong enough to endure the disaster that divorce proceedings will bring. The legal community is not aware and has failed to educate itself about the high conflict inherit with these mixed neurological marriages. For whatever the reason, these women will continue to need support while they try to make their relationships work, even in the short term or when embarking alone on a new life direction.

We bring what we can to each person who wants to remain in their marriage, but most of us have given up on preserving it, having tried everything, and came to the realization it is futile to save a relationship that in the most practical sense is not one. Since the normal partner is the only one capable of changing and they have tried that time and again, the outlook is dim. We were married to men who allowed us to wander through mazes fraught with confusion, pain, and misleading images and were happy to let us struggle with the self-doubt. They never took responsibility for the misunderstandings or for the pain they inflicted and never owned up to their contribution for the failure. We reached a point where all we want to do is to stay sane and alive—happiness remains a distant dream. Each of us has at one time or another felt the only escape from the "hell" we live in is our own death, it seems like the only exit.

The women in my support group knew of my intention to write this book and have consented to allow me use their stories as long as their anonymity is protected and I do that without reservation.

One woman told us of the time she and her husband went to family counseling where her "left brained" spouse used his intellectual, professional and articulate faculties to "snow" the therapist and "talked the talk." She sat there as the mute partner while she witnessed her Aspie spouse monopolize the conversation and manipulate the therapist into believing that he was in fact Mr. Wonderful, Mr. Sweetness and Light, who was always trying to do the right thing (abiding by the rules), but she was uncooperative, and thwarted his sincere desire to have a healthy relationship (control her). He wanted the therapist to see his logical explanation for their turmoil (all her fault) and understand why he (the perfect one) was unable to facilitate a marriage with her (the nut case). She said on the ride back home she knew it was hopeless. He had assaulted her on several occasions and when the police were called, she was the one who had to spend the night in jail because "ole left brain" could use convincing logical arguments and all she had were small bruises, tears and anger. Women use emotions to voice their side of the story, men use logic. We have been conditioned to believe the ring of truth resides exclusively in logic as opposed to the belief that emotions bear the truth, too. When men cry we are moved, when children cry we respond, but when women cry, we are manipulative.

In AS marriages this is the reverse; these men use logic and condescension for manipulation, and women use emotional outbursts as cries for understanding and need of support. This is the standard irresolvable dilemma we face every day—credibility.

This is not an isolated illustration of the strife and frustration which haunts women in Aspie marriages, this is the norm. And when a couple goes to court for divorce and child custody, here is where the conflict gets ramped up and ugly.

One wife and the mother of two small children is a family law attorney who is currently trying to divorce her Aspie spouse. Since he in his thirties he escaped professional diagnosis—but not hers—she knows through her own experience and research that he is on the spectrum (wives are the best diagnosticians for this disorder).

She knows he lacks core parenting skills and can only parent with her guidance and support. A familiar Aspie characteristic is if once shown how to do something, he immediately becomes an expert on the subject and thinks he is the Father of the Year. When he "helps" with the children, she needs to check the bath water so it isn't too hot for the children. She can look at her sick child and decide if a doctor's visit or hospital visit is appropriate, and she can determine if her child is hurting or in pain, or just tired and hungry, all the subtle signs mothers intuitively look for when assessing their children's health and well being, the vague signs AS spouses miss and are unable to respond to appropriately.

She is upset and worried about his aggressive pursuit of shared custody for their two year old and five year old. He doesn't want the divorce (it creates a disruption in the force, a bad thing when involved with an Aspie) and is using the custody issue to manipulate her into staying in the marriage. She knows she is legally restricted from requesting the court to address his disorder and must comply with any decision it makes, all the time knowing she is endangering her children and their welfare by placing them in his care. We have prayed about this and I continue to support her via phone as often as she needs it. It is imperative I remind her that she is a strong, loving, intelligent woman for her to maintain her faith in herself. During this divorce, her self-doubts are off the wall—what a needless waste of her energy. We all need this so much in our lives and are so appreciative when someone sees this need and offers to validate us.

Family court professionals have little knowledge of ASD (Asperger's Syndrome Disorder) or education in the area of divorce and child custody cases in families affected by ASD. They must learn about the limitations of the ASD parent or in some cases, parents, and the trauma to the overstressed, normal parent when general legal rulings are applied to these non-standard cases. A "one size fits all" custody arrangement cannot be applied to the children in these failed marriages because of the neurological differences demonstrated by the affected parent and the resulting behaviors which may be detrimental physically and emotionally to the children. Anything short of an in-depth investigation by child advocates or DSS should be considered irresponsible and culpable.

I want to make the case for these families by way of suggesting to women who are planning to file for divorce that they make it clear to their attorney they are married to a partner who is on the spectrum and prepare for conflict from the ASD partner. It would be beneficial to take a copy of the article about divorce presented by FAAAS, Inc., *Autism in Children and Parents: Unique Considerations for Family Court Professionals*, by Sheila Jennings and present it to your legal representative. Perhaps over time these professionals will create a database to be used to establish an accurate statistic for the divorce rate among AS individuals as litigants, which is currently estimated at 80%. Establishing a legal specialization for ASD families should be paramount as well as beneficial.

The tragedy here is these women are not by their nature women who are angry or have anger management problems; they find themselves simmering with this negative emotion after years of subjugating themselves to childish, demanding men who never consider their basic feeling of being a living, breathing, needing human being.

When we have conflicts in the marriage, we get very little support from family, friends, or professionals; there is a natural and understandable hesitancy on the part of these "outsiders" to assume what is being asked is to take sides and that's not the case. What others believe to be a normal and isolated domestic spat is actually a lifestyle insidiously and incrementally constructed over time by the insensitive behavior and demands of the Aspie upon the normal partner. And because the Aspie looks normal and speaks in a logical and often a highly professional way, the light of suspicion is usually focused on what appears to be an irrational, anxious, highly emotional woman who is merely asking for the validation she is not crazy or delusional. Regrettably, sympathy is usually and erroneously granted exclusively to the aardvark.

When this misjudgment occurs (and it often does), outsiders have unknowingly undermined the very support system the Aspie needs to survive by further weakening the normal spouse's need for validation and support to keep both parties afloat.

We all agree we could scream when our feelings are misinterpreted and negated by casual observers. If we dare share information about our "weird" marriages to outsiders, we are usually told all husbands do these infuriating things, making us want to tear our hair out and scream, "Yeah, well, all men don't do everything my husband does, walk in my shoes and then get back to me."

The biggest problem we have to face in our culture is the lack of empathy and the recognition of real pain and the sense of loss over losing a real husband we never truly had. We only empathize when there is a grave or death certificate. Widows are entitled, but not divorcees, or Aspie spouses.

I look into the eyes of these loving, smart and strong women who are wounded and have the look of a deer caught in the headlights as a permanent expression etched into the landscape of their lovely, tired faces. No woman should have to endure the cruelty of abuse or neglect, whether it comes from alcohol, drugs, domestic violence or Asperger's Syndrome. Our wounds and scars are much deeper and will remain untreated until the rest of the world gains some awareness and insight into the difficult lives we live.

We share a list of maladies, physical and mental: migraines, digestive problems, hypertension, weight gain or loss, ME (myalgic-encephalomyelitis), and a compromised immune system, anything from colds to cancer. We know we'll probably die long before our spouses if with nothing else, but exhaustion and neglect. No one has done any suicidal studies on our population to date; I imagine it happens more often than one may think.

The ages of these women span from the late twenties into the eighties, as do their spouses, and they look exhausted beyond their years.

Everyone at the meeting tries to name one or two things that are positive about their spouses; it is the most difficult part of our meeting. For the meager number of positives there are dozens of negatives to reclaim them.

Some are glad their husbands have good paying jobs—at least some financial security helps sweeten the burgeoning list of difficulties. But most would rather have less, much less materially and have a normal spouse who recognizes their existence and contributions and can show it. Some appreciate the fidelity even if it is not intentional, but probably situational—no one else would want him! Several have even wished some woman would come along and entice their spouse away so they wouldn't have to deal with their puerile, life smothering obsessions. We are possessions who belong to them in perpetuity, like a parent who should never leave. Every time I asked Clay for a divorce his excuses ran from, "We can't afford it," and "I don't have any friends," to stubborn silence.

We even talk about our sex life, at least those who have one. Their sense of humor about this subject is honest and unexpected. Some of us have been married before and have a comparative which comes in handy for describing the difference in the sex life of normal men and Aspies. We were all shocked to learn we were virtually going to bed with the same man. Aspies don't caress, they grope—something akin to a child grabbing for candy from a ruptured Piñata. It's a business transaction, serious and unemotional. They've all read the same manual and proceed accordingly, attempting to frantically push all the buttons at the same time expecting a gumball to come rolling out of a slot. It can also be uncomfortable because these guys are single minded and want to get it over with as soon as possible and may inflict some damage during the course of the proceedings. We all agree this is not the style of love making we had in mind or experienced in our past lives. The act leaves much to be desired and some prefer to become celibate wives if they have a choice, some of us don't, yours truly included. It hurts to know I have lost my last chance to have a satisfying love life with a normal, loving and expressive man.

With an Aspie there is no pillow talk, compliments about your performance and no declarations of undying love. Money left on the dresser along with a business card would feel more appropriate.

Some of these younger women had no premarital experience and were shocked to hear what they had missed: seduction, arousal, and earth shaking satisfaction and an emotional connection.

One attractive, professional young woman said she was afraid to leave her spouse because she didn't think she could find another man. Sad to think she feels she had to stay in an unhappy marriage for fear of being alone. The truth is we are alone in these relationships anyway. I listened to their stories and heard mine echoing repeatedly in their voices and felt their tears on my face.

Often I see ads about Autism and see only the face of a child, but I know the public is missing the other faces in the Autism family album—the spouses.

## CHAPTER 20

*"Human history becomes more and more a race between education and catastrophe."*

—H.G. Wells

There are also many women who are not only spouses of Aspies, but are also mothers of children on the spectrum. These women can be overwhelmed with not only the daily care of their children, but a spouse on the spectrum. Whether it's Classical Autism (CA), High Functioning Autism (HFA), Asperger's Syndrome (AS), or grouped together as autism spectrum disorders or ASD disabilities; care for these children is not simple or cheap. It usually entails the coordination of teams of child development specialists: physicians, occupational therapists, social skills therapists, behavioral specialists, speech therapists, medical assessors, tutors, psychotherapists, autism support group facilitators, parent-training teachers, and any family members who are capable and willing to give them a break. Then there is the cost estimated at $3.2 million USD over the course of a lifetime for one child (some families have more than a single child requiring these services), and for society, treating these children is estimated at an annual cost of $85 billion USD. It's expensive and time consuming.

Caring for some AS offspring can be the least complicated of the three to manage, time and cost wise, particularly if the parents are aware of the disorder and have been given insight and instruction to avert any learning disabilities or behavioral problems.

The prevalence of Autism is shown to be anywhere from 1 in 250 persons, or 1 in 144 or 166; these numbers bounce all over the place and create confusion. To understand what is happening requires an explanation of how statisticians use this data.

First we must understand these numbers reflect different values: 1 in 250 represents Asperger's Syndrome, 1 in 166 through 1 in 144 represents Classical Autism, High Functioning Autism, or it can be an inclusion of all three. Since the presence of any one of these disorders on the spectrum is called autism, it is difficult to know which degree is in question. We've been alerted almost weekly through the media about the explosion of autism in this country (as well as around the globe), but since the level of care and cost differs somewhat along the spectrum, we would do well to ask what type of autism is being cited in these statistics.

Since many of these individuals require lifetime care and financial support, it is important to make the point that if the prevalence is 1 in 144, the other 143 will be required to support the "one," either financially or professionally.

Asperger's Syndrome has only been on the radar in this country since 1994, ten years after Lorna Wing, a psychiatrist in the UK, coined the term. And ever since it was entered in the DSM IV (Diagnostic and Statistical Manual of Mental Disorders), its statistical data has annually climbed off the charts.

Many claim that this is the result of the new diagnostic criteria, which may have snatched individuals previously diagnosed with other Pervasive Development Disorders (PPDs) and placed them under the autism umbrella. Still others believe that the increase is due to an actual "head" count. Many states in the US have seen increases since the tracking of autism during the period of 1993 through 2001: 23 states have had an increase of 1000%; another 15 states had increases of between 500% and 900%.

Worldwide, the rate of autism among children has risen 800%.

Much has been written and documented about autism and the most highly theorized and controversial aspect of this disorder is its cause. People want to know where it comes from and how do people "get" it?

There are many theories, and to date, none are considered definitive. The more popular theories offered by researchers are those that maintain and support the notion that the cause is from various environmental sources creating a toxicity occurring during pregnancy and transferred from the mother to the fetus. This remains the most widely accepted underlying factor that runs in tandem with every other theory.

The theory which is the more widely publicized by activist parents groups is the belief that childhood inoculations are responsible for the upsurge in "regressive" autism which occurs in children up to the age of four and who were perceived to be developmentally normal until they receive their MMR and DPT vaccinations.

Parents with children on the spectrum are convinced that either the mercury in these vaccines was responsible for their child's disorder, or it was the new vaccine guidelines dictated by the CDC mandating as many as thirty (plus or minus) inoculations to be given by the age of eighteen to twenty-four months, and I agree this does seem excessive.

The media covers many reports a year on this topic, but five major medical studies have concluded this is not the case since the elimination of thimerosal (mercury) from childhood vaccines in 2001, and the incident of autism keeps climbing. But these parents are convinced the very inoculations used to safeguard their children from horrible and potentially fatal diseases are the most popularly suspected culprit triggering the disorder. We do know there is a genetic factor and in Asperger's Syndrome and HFA it's hereditary, probably caused by a gene contributed from both parents.

I personally know it's hereditary since I live with four generations of AS. I've heard other women repeat stories about this type of family history. I also know if you have a child with an AS partner, you will have one or potentially all of your children on the spectrum. So it appears if you don't want to have children with HFA or AS—you may want to find another mate.

HFA manifests itself as the ultimate "geek" archetype, with highly distinguishable physical and behavioral characteristics.

The familiar image most people have is of the nerdy guy with the thick eyeglasses, the pocket protector, awkward and clumsy body movements, and he may be the science whiz in high school. To listen to him you would think this guy invented every computer language in existence and all its associated technology—and he did, or at least someone like him did. He was the kid most likely to be bullied or on the receiving end of adolescents' most humiliating of hazing practices—the toilet swirly. He is going to show up at every Star Trek convention—in costume and speaking Klingon (invented language of aliens in the TV series Star Trek). He collects vintage comic books and his life is defined by outer space: astronomy, astrophysics, science fiction/fantasy and the ethernet. As a rule, this guy doesn't get married unless he makes a boat load of money and can convince some girl he has some potential to be adequately socialized. Although, all Aspies are geeks, not all geeks are Aspies—a distinction which needs to made so as not to stampede several hundred thousand people to diagnostic centers.

The best example of the HFA, geek personality is "Sheldon," the character on "The Big Bang Theory," who is tall, lean, asexual, emotionally immature, nerdish and exasperating. I get concerned when the media comes up with reality shows like, "The Beauty and the Geek," attempting to make a love match between two people who are destined to clash cultures and egos, resulting in disaster for both parties—love does not necessarily conquer all.

These guys at their level of social disability are readily noticeable and are quickly labeled "weird," whereas men with AS like Clay, the ultra-functioning member of the spectrum, present a challenge to the casual observer. Although Clay has subtle impairment in the areas of emotional and social interactions, his intellect obscures his disorder from the outside world and professionals and, most disturbingly, from me, his spouse, who went bonkers attempting to figure out what in the hell was wrong with this man. To give an example of the exasperation I experienced living with Clay and expose a well kept secret: the technical manuals that come with many products, the ones that will have you tearing out your hair while inventing new and obscene expletives: they are written by guys like Clay. Well crafted instructions that sadistically fail to instruct clearly are logical but incomprehensible. Try living with someone who communicates like that—all the time.

Even if a woman recognizes these weird fellows and avoids them in the social scene of dating or marriage, they are out there procreating. One recently shocking development has affected some women who have chosen to be artificially inseminated via sperm banks and they are discovering sperm donors may be on the spectrum.

The Associated Press article, "Sperm Donations Under Scrutiny," dated August, 2006, written by Kim Nguyen, told the story of a woman who had conceived a child from sperm donated by a mystery man known only as Donor 3066 from the California Cryobank. Her daughter and at least six other children by different mothers were fathered by the same donor. She discovered that four of the seven were diagnosed as being on the spectrum. So even if a woman is highly selective about a sperm donor for her baby, there may be some anonymous Aspie out there fathering these children.

Scientists have as yet been unable to isolate and identify the autism gene, which could one day be used to determine the genetic outcome of the unborn.

Although Cryobank put Donor 3066 on "restricted" status, women could still use his sperm, but were warned that problems could arise with their children.

Cryobank issued a statement saying that they have their donors fill out an exhaustive medical and personal history application that includes three generations.

However, if these men haven't been diagnosed with AS or HFA or do have it but wish to not make a disclosure (you can't hold up a plastic specimen cup of semen and see sperm swimming around wearing glasses and pocket protectors), then these applications are useless in preventing the use of spectrum sperm.

The dream of having a "genius," a brilliant scientist, or a famous musician father a child appeals to women who want exceptionally bright progeny; it is not unheard of for these women to seek sperm candidates who are above average intelligence to guarantee themselves a superlative offspring. But, as presented in this article, it's not necessarily safe to assume a "test tube" father offers any greater certainty of healthy, smart issue than the guy who lives down the street and pumps gas for a living.

Another of the theories about the cause of autism is "assortative mating." This theory is based on the belief that two people who share common traits and interests will marry and create a genetic overload of autistic traits endowing their children with spectrum disorders.

The December 2001 article appearing in Wired 9:12, "The Geek Syndrome," written by Steve Silberman, goes into great detail in explanation of this theory.

Silberman explains how certain high tech and R&D corridors around the country (Silicon Valley, Bricktown, N.J., RTP, N.C.) hire many geekish engineers, scientists, and computer programmers, male and female, who, unlike the rest of us who randomly mate in a crap-shoot fashion based only on physical and emotional compatibility, are more or less genetically preordained to play out their predisposition to autism with similarly structured mates and produce little geeks.

A 2006 article, "Parents' Marriage Choice May Lead to Autism," written by Roger Highfield, Science Editor of Telegraph.co.uk, cites new studies by Professor Baron-Cohen, a clinical psychologist with an impressive body of work in autism at Cambridge University, in which he divided the world into two distinctive mind sets: Systemizers and Empathizers. People on the spectrum, like engineers and computer programmers, reside in the systemizers camp, and the rest of us are categorized as empathizers.

I think the Baron-Cohen theory leaves no room for the mainstream mentality the majority of us who are considered normal are utilizing. We integrate both hemispheres of our brains making us systemizers and empathizers and survive rather well employing the combined functions of our brains as feeling and thinking human beings.

Professor Baron-Cohen further claims the rise in autism could be driven by the ease of assortative mating. Given the new mobility and rise of employment prospects of systemizers in the computer industry and the addition of women in these "geek" fields of mathematics and engineering, as well as medicine and other scientific and academic enclaves, these men and women are in daily contact with each other and a mutual recognition of shared interests and attraction is inevitable.

Brain scan studies have shown of the mothers and fathers of children with autism, the mothers have a masculinized pattern of brain activity, suggesting they are strong systemizers.

In his paper, "Is Asperger's Syndrome/High Functioning Autism a Disability?", Professor Baron-Cohen uses a recent study that found out of 1,000 families, 28.4 children had ASD or AS and had at least one relative (father or grandfather) who was an engineer.

In a survey of students at Cambridge University who were studying either the sciences or humanities and were asked about family history, the students in the science group showed a six-fold increase in the rate of autism in their families and this was specific to autism (not schizophrenia, Down Syndrome, language delay, or manic depression).

The professor also makes the case for science and technology, the talents of people with AS is a boon and asks, "Is it a disability?"

He doesn't think within the context of computer programming or scientific research where intense focus on detail is highly desirable and necessary, that this autistic trait is a disability or handicap, but sees it as a talent. I agree with his statement. I saw this same dedicated attention to detail in Clay, and knew this particular trait was an advantage for him in his career as a computer systems programmer. I know this talent serves him well in his occupation but is of little or no value in a marital relationship.

I agree within the given parameters of science and computer technology, AS is not a disability. But in the areas of social interaction, specifically marriage, the AS personality is at a disadvantage and should be considered, "highly limited."

I feel it would be a hard reality to face a narrow and neurologically limited lifestyle. Yet as I read the posts on Aspie chat forums, I came to realize these people are happy with their lives and eschew the efforts of "curbies" (those who are trying to find a cure for autism). They prefer their world of narrow self-interests and resent the attitude of NTs who want to change or cure them. They would rather have the whole world function as they do, believing, as Mr. Spock would say, "It's logical."

They chafe under the burdens placed on them by NTs to make eye contact or change any of the inherent characteristics of the Aspie personality and lifestyle. But why wouldn't they prefer a world where they are sheltered and supported and can make above average salaries, have flexible work schedules, contained environments, and are thought of as geniuses?

We have already seen the influence of how AS preferences impact on our culture; we email instead of talking on the phone or writing letters by hand, preferring the anonymity of the computer. Aspies can remain anonymous and persuade by the written word rather than having to use eye contact, body language or any other social conventions to convey their thoughts. This brings me to one last theory—the parents of children on the spectrum met online.

## CHAPTER 21

*"We read to know we are not alone."*

—C.S. Lewis

Although the wife of an Aspie is unhappy, the Aspie is disproportionately happy and contented compared to his frazzled spouse. He has few physical needs other than food and sleep, and his only other requirement is uninterrupted time to pursue his "special" interests and to control his environment; these controlling mechanisms keep harmony within the "force" but are also the greatest unrelenting drain on his energy causing him to often erupt into rages when disturbed. Sounds pretty simple and on the surface it is, but once you add another person or persons to this equation and the frictional sparks begin to fly, they're going land squarely on someone else—spouse and/or children.

If a woman can wrap her mind around the image of a moderately sedate but on occasion a highly volatile adolescent male who prefers to stay in his room and enjoy his particular interests and who should only be called upon to come down to eat meals with no other demands on him for fulfilling her needs or helping with domestic maintenance, then she can understand the basic requirements for the care and feeding of an Aspie.

The problems between these two partners occur during the emergence of opposing expectations: she is expecting a husband who is a helpmate, a soul mate, a protector and provider, a supporter and comforter for her physical and emotional needs, and she willingly expects to reciprocate all these things. He on the other hand has an entirely different expectation: a sexually undemanding "playmate," a social tutor, interpreter and a mama—someone who will, on demand, be there to share his all consuming interests, indulge him and bestow adoration while contributing an inexhaustible amount of energy toward his happiness and comfort. Remember, these people are unabashedly self-centered, and if you profess your love for them, they assume these demands are not excessive or unreasonable. After all, mom did all of this and she thinks he's wonderful and God's gift to mankind, because he's sooo smart!

Oh, how we cater to the selfish demands of genius (although AS is not an automatic certification of genius, many have an average I.Q.).

Many women are going to scratch their heads and say, "Gee, he sounds like my husband. I thought all men were like this." Unfortunately, most men do have a lot in common with the Aspie personality since most men are left brain dominant and share many Aspie traits. But there is a huge difference; the majority of men can choose to use the right hemisphere of their brain and access the positives this lovely twin of the left hemisphere offers to garner and demonstrate the appropriate feelings in order to bring harmony and romance back into the marriage. These men know what they need to do and say to attract the wife back into their camp for the contentment of both. If they don't, at least they have the good sense to ask a friend what to do and follow through. In other words, they are capable of negotiating a resolution for the purpose of keeping the peace.

I once bought Clay a book, "Romance for Dummies," it's the only book in his collection of over several hundred tomes he has never read—right book, wrong dummy. This action alone should indicate to any woman, "Honey, he's just not that into you."

With clocklike precision he would bring me flowers or a gift for my birthday, Valentine's Day, and our wedding anniversary. He would ask, without much enthusiasm, if I wanted to go out for dinner. Dinners out with Clay were excruciatingly awkward and boring. He had nothing to say unless it was his normal daily report—news, weather, etc. And that was the extent of it—no romance, no sexual overtures, no sweet endearments. Now this may sound like I'm some high maintenance biddy who was never satisfied with her husband's effort, but actually it is far from the real "me." I would have been deeply touched and thrilled by simple shared moments where we gazed into each other's eyes, laid sheltered in each other's arms and talked about our dreams of the future, and laughed or cried about the past; we never in over twenty-five years wrote our story. In my life with Clay, the saddest legacy his disorder left me was the absence of happy, heartwarming memories; the ones that keep you cozy and comforted on a lonely, cold night. Any warm memories of us don't exist—there is only a blank slate of time where nothing is written with love on the walls of the heart—an eternal hollowness for my soul to wander through, never able to furnish.

I was still learning the hard way (the only available method most of the time), about the strange inner workings of this weird animal who was curled up in his burrow and married to me.

Aspies see the world in black and white; we see the world in black and white and shades of gray. Normal folk and Aspies are not opposites; we all possess the same portion of gray cells, which can quantify and analyze information, but this is predominately the Aspie's only system operating at full capacity. We share the same intellectual traits, but for us, these cold and stringent robotic talents are mitigated by the many influences of the gentler side of the brain, specifically the empathetic, imagining, and spiritual half. It has the ability to smooth and refine the sharply piercing edges of the human mind and its resulting actions into a softer, more flexible and reciprocating process, which transforms human discord into a life-affirming and supportive social order.

From the beginning of my marriage to Clay, I couldn't see or understand all of the differences separating and preventing us from melding our opposing mindsets. We were trying to independently adapt to the alien demands set forth by the other. I know it affected my health and my sense of well-being in a manner I could have never expected. I was disappointed to discover I was not in the kind of relationship I had dreamed of for so many years, but found my life was filled with unpleasant surprises, mind numbing revelations. I tried to figure out what I was contributing to the ongoing upheaval and confusion and was also blaming myself for our misunderstandings and my reactions to his behavior. In order for me to accurately formulate a perception of Clay, I had to use both lenses of my brain to integrate the contrasting images of him. I needed both sides of my brain, and then some, in an attempt to understand this strange entity, when in the final analysis, this was futile. Only the description of AS could bring him into total focus. By nature, he resided in his left brain and any interaction between us required him to drag me kicking and screaming (neurologically speaking) over to his dominant side, and this recurring action over time, I believe, finally resulted in my developing migraines a year and a half after we married which continue to this day. He controls conversations by keeping them in a logical context where he has the home court advantage and is most comfortable. Now, I understand what I was doing wrong—I was being normal, but before I arrived at this discovery, I contracted a syndrome of my own.

In Greek mythology, King Priam, the ruler of Troy had a daughter, Cassandra. Her beauty attracted the attention of Apollo and he initially gave her the gift of prophecy, but when she refused his advances, he placed a curse on her ensuring no one would believe her warnings. She had the knowledge of future events but couldn't change them or convince others of the validity of her predictions—thus creating the Cassandra Syndrome.

Some psychologists apply the Cassandra metaphor to individuals who have experienced physical and emotional suffering as the result of distressing personal perceptions and are disbelieved as they attempt to share the cause of their suffering with others.

Jean Shinoda-Bolen, Clinical Professor of Psychiatry at the University of California, published an essay on the god Apollo. She compiled a psychological profile of the "Cassandra Woman" whom she referred to as someone suffering, as in the relationship between Apollo and Cassandra—a dysfunctional relationship with an "Apollo man."

She describes the negative Apollonic influence as: "Individuals who resemble Apollo have difficulties that are related to emotional distance, such as communication problems, and the inability to be intimate... Rapport with another person is hard for the Apollo man. He prefers to access (or judge) the situation or the person from a distance, not knowing that he must 'get close up'—be vulnerable and empathic—in order to truly know someone else..."

Shinoda-Bolen wrote this paper in 1989, five years before the DMS IV set forth the diagnostic criteria for Asperger's Syndrome, but she managed to accurately nail the AS male in her paper as the negative Apollo archetype.

In 1988, Jungian analyst Laurie Layton Schapira explored the "Cassandra Complex" stating: "What the Cassandra woman sees is something dark and painful that may not be apparent on the surface of things or that objective facts do not corroborate. She may envision a negative or unexpected outcome; or something which would be difficult to deal with; or a truth which others, especially authority figures, would not accept. In her frightened, ego-less state, the Cassandra woman may blurt out what she sees, perhaps with the unconscious hope that others might be able to make some sense of it. But to them her words sound meaningless, disconnected and blown out of all proportion."

This was what I experienced with each visit to a therapist, with or without Clay, but certainly with a more profound and discrediting outcome on my behalf when he accompanied me. Mr. Brilliant or Mr. Non-threatening sitting beside me with his calm and controlled demeanor in the presence of a professional brought out the best in him and the worst in me. It was a "no-win" contest creating even greater anxiety and depression for me. It was a vicious cycle of misdiagnosis for us both.

I had to let all of this go to overcome the imprisonment of Clay's disorder. The isolation and loneliness were enough to cause severe depression, and I had to use my meager reserves of strength and resolve to avoid letting it completely pull me under.

I decided to get out and join a local social club, one involving couples. I jumped in, cleaned up Clay, and off we went. At first, all went rather well and he seemed to look forward to the dinners out and would always find some willing, unsuspecting soul who would tolerate his self-centric interests. Although I enjoyed getting out, meeting people and doing something other than sitting at home alone with dunderhead, I soon became uncomfortable with the atmosphere of other couples joking and kidding with their spouses and demonstrating affection for each other. It made me painfully aware of what I was missing in the marriage and it hurt—deeply. I grew even unhappier with Clay; the contrast between him and the other husbands was so obvious to everyone except Clay. I felt left out. I was at the prom with my brother.

On one occasion, a new female friend saw Clay place his hand on my shoulder and commented how she thought this was a demonstration of affection. I had to ruin her interpretation of his gesture and tell her Clay always did that when he felt insecure in social gatherings.

Anyone in Clay's presence would initially assume he is an intelligent, polite and friendly man and normal in every aspect. Clay does well on the job and loves his work, and on rare occasions meets with his co-workers for drinks at day's end. Naturally, casual observers don't see what I have seen or experienced and find it difficult to believe that I would have any legitimate reason for not being deliriously satisfied with this man and if he were my son, yes, but he's not.

Asperger's is not recent or new, it has probably been around for over a thousand years. Many famous people are on the spectrum, for a look at the list, just type "Famous Aspies" into the search engine of choice and prepare to be amazed at all the Nobel Prize winners.

I hope by reading my story, other women who share this bizarre world of AS may feel comforted to know someday others will learn of our hidden life and come to understand and hopefully lend support or at the very least listen. Education is the first step toward understanding, followed by the acceptance of the many alternate realities that reside right next door.

## CHAPTER 22

*"He was . . . My noon, my midnight, my talk, my song.
I thought that love would last forever : I was wrong."*
—W.H. Auden

The journey I undertook twenty-five years ago with Clay has been fraught with the lingering images of nightmares. I was ill prepared for this excursion into the realm of Asperger's and was equally ill equipped for dealing with the devastating impact it presented in my life. I had only one defensive weapon for combating this overwhelming and confusing adversary: my all consuming desire to identify and disarm it, I succeeded in only one of these goals. The one question people invariably ask me, "Why did you stay?" There is no simple answer. It makes me uncomfortable when presented with this understandable query because, first, it feels like an indictment of my intelligence in the face of the many complaints I had about Clay and his bizarre actions, and second, staying with him made me look like an imbecilic masochist—the jury is still out on both. In my defense, I was always thrown off balance by the contrasting images of this smart man/child who could convince through rational speech, and then confuse by immature behavior. He was at times the intelligent, sane one making me doubt my judgment until the weird behavior kicked in allowing me to briefly embrace the belief that I was the only rational one. He could quite comfortably and without conscience allow me to run in circles trying to make sense of this warped reality. I couldn't determine who was nuts and who wasn't and he was cruelly content to let me think it was I. We both couldn't be normal at the same time without negating the other's true nature; we couldn't co-exist with opposing and colliding mentalities. I lived within an Escher drawing trying to establish my equilibrium in this disorienting rendering of divided planes—"Are you really sure a floor can't also be a ceiling?" To maintain my well-being, he would have to go; to maintain his, I would have to acquiesce, and crumble I did. I stayed because the self-doubt and low self-esteem induced by his AS made his world for short intervals appear more logical than mine, although it never felt comfortable or legitimate.

I remember the day we were en route to our wedding, *something* made me ask him not just once, but three times to turn around and take me home—that something was my inner voice and I allowed him to convince me to ignore it.

My life followed the winding plot line of a suspenseful mystery, with hundreds of sharp twists and turns just when you begin to think you know who the culprit is all the clues and evidence lead you to another red herring before discovering the true villain; obviously AS is the only culprit here.

As I said several times in my story, I never really perceived Clay's actions as being intentionally mean-spirited, but the effects of his behavior became impossible for me to abide; even when I understood the provenance of his actions, it was unacceptable and felt life-threatening.

When I initially read the indicators for Asperger's Syndrome . . . "they have communication problems and lack empathy," I found those disturbing words on the page disconnected from the flesh and emotion. I had to bring substance to those printed characters in order to give them weight, mass and a pulse before applying them to Clay and my life. Words are marvelous representatives, but when I read about AS without the context of real life experiences I couldn't understand exactly what they meant or how it applied to us. An example: "they don't like change," what kind of change—the weather, clean underwear, or oil, what? I was able to parse the applicable meaning of "change" by observing Clay and came to understand it meant an interruption of his concentration or the modification of his environment in any manner—like rearranging the furniture. I incarnated these printed "symptoms," dressed them in clothes

# THE AARDVARK'S WIFE

and sat them down inside my home, where they became all too real and painfully familiar.

I wanted to convey to a reader how these traits and their subsequent actions skewed the reality of my life and how it made me feel and react. I wanted to share how living without empathy became wounding and isolating.

I often hear people, especially teachers, discussing a loss of empathy in society and the classroom, and wonder to what they should attribute this slowly disappearing value. I think it is obvious when studying the impact of AS traits on industry, technology, science and society. And as the prevalence of AS increases, this admirable quality decreases. We continue to lose empathy, but gain another step forward in technology with each passing generation.

When, years ago, I moved out of our bedroom, finally accepting the grim truth that I was married to a man who didn't appear to want or need me as a wife. Clay never asked why or tried to persuade me to return to his bed. I cried myself to sleep for more nights than I can count, and became his "housemate," never breaching the unspoken contract that defined our stressed and meaningless relationship. I wasn't married nor was I single. I existed in a social limbo, never belonging anywhere. I haven't made love in eighteen years. Friends often ask me why I didn't have an affair—I wouldn't break my marriage vows and in the light of my track record with *two* husbands, I don't trust myself to find someone who would be willing to restore my faith in relationships—it's too much to ask of anyone.

Being lonely in a marriage because you have no one to talk to or never feeling understood makes for an empty home. Having no shared commitment to a dream makes an empty, cold bed. I had all the responsibilities of marriage and none of the rewards. I worked, cleaned house, cooked and carried the burdens of life's disappointments alone. I made the sacrifices and compromises marriage requires when two people share a space and a life. I continued to look forward to the day it would be reciprocated in some manner and accepted the cruel hope of believing that someday, somehow, it would become a real marriage. I know that the loneliness of being single and alone and not having anyone to talk to, and no sense of being understood also means there is no one standing between me and the life I want to give myself. There are two kinds of loneliness and the kind experienced in the presence of another is the worst, it reverberates with rejection.

Clay lives his life cylindrically and I live mine spherically; he is restricted to this self-serving lifestyle of special ego-centric interests and acts according to this particular mindset. I, on the other hand, want and need to live in the way my heart and soul require to be contented and fulfilled. I want to reach out and embrace people, learn new skills, and be touched with affection without having to ask, and to be *pleasantly* surprised once in a while. When I fight with someone I don't want it to end in an impasse with the stomping out of the room never to be resolved; I want to make up and heal. I want to share dreams. I want to laugh. I want to cry, not from pain, but because I am moved. I want to create good memories, and I want to do all these things with a soul mate. I have been starved for all these many wonderful, human and spiritual gifts and I know Clay can't deliver them. I am truly sorry that he couldn't be the *one* because I think without AS he would have been the best!

I have the benefit of experience with the disorder which insidiously robbed me of a husband and a happy, fulfilling marriage. I can't restore my life to an earlier status, but I am willing to offer support to the women who are still in these marriages filled with confusing signals and hurtful consequences who need to be comforted by knowing there is a life outside of AS.

So many women I have spoken with have the idea they can never leave for fear "he" will have no one to take care of him, they won't venture far from home for any length of time to explore their interests, or reclaim a life left behind at the altar. They believe their AS spouse incapable of caring for himself; this is half true, they can survive alone, although they will always require some degree of shepherding. It is a common misconception cementing many women in the marriages they wish to dissolve. If left alone he will immediately go out and find another "mama"; some AS men and women marry three, four or five times searching for a shepherd, and that is precisely what their next spouse will become.

I hope to raise awareness and rally the mental health and legal communities to recognize the plight of so many and bring a new, enlightened sensitivity to the predicament of AS spouses in the practice of their individual professions.

I believe training therapists for the treatment of Cassandra Syndrome would greatly alleviate the emotional and mental confusion experienced by women living in marriages with AS men. I can't empathize enough the despair and pain of having no one to relate the devastating experiences of these marriages. I hope to see the expansion of support group networks across the country for the purpose of giving voice to those who need validation and guidance. The UK and Australia have demonstrated a far more progressive attitude for these social services.

I don't personally advocate for a marriage between two diverse neurological partners, but I sincerely hope any woman contemplating marriage to the "quirky" man reading or on the computer in the next room will take the initiative and learn more about AS through reading and listening to the experiences by other veterans of this "marital" disorder rather than learning through raw experience. And if indeed the evidence proves that this very smart, but strange person you fell in love with does have Asperger's, please make the effort to locate a counselor with strong AS expertise; it could make a world of difference in the quality of your life—forewarned is forearmed.

I want to make it clear that people on the spectrum are not evil people, and are trying their best to be good spouses and parents, but as the saying goes they do march to a different tune. I want to make potential NT spouses aware that there is going to be a mountain of obstacles to overcome and it will require patience and tolerance on your part to make this type of marriage work. I am sorry to disappoint those who thought I would be able to impart some magical solution to the question of how to thrive in these relationships, I cannot. My only advice is to accept it for what it is, understand the impossibility of change, and pray for strength and support. I will, however, say that if you decide to leave please know that I and many others do understand and feel deeply for your loss.

## ACKNOWLEDGEMENTS

As with almost anything in life, we rarely do much without help. I was blessed to have had many wonderful and qualified people to not only encourage me, but who were willing to help "row" my boat and correct the occasional veering off course.

When I lost sight of my destination, they were there lighting flares and waving me on.

First, I want to thank (a small word to represent the volumes of sincere appreciation I feel) all the great gals in my writer's group. These women are not only accomplished in their professional careers, but are precisely what the definition of "friend" should be. Grace Rowlson, therapist and writer, who never let me say, "I quit!" or allowed me to do so. She possesses a unique and uncanny ability to detect B.S., wherever she sees it, particularly on paper. Thanks, Grace for keeping me on track. Stephanie Smith, Ph.D., who has an intuitive and dedicated approach to memoir writing, her insight and critical eye taught me to stand back and look and then look again. She's a teacher and writer. Denise Sherman, journalist, artist and writer, her artistic spirit and realistic treatment of subject matter brings whimsy and fact together in an unforgettable wedding of phrases. These amazing and supportive women brought their sharply honed skill for critique to my work and prevented it from disappearing into a shoe box.

I must also thank my friend and fellow writer, Gurpreet Jawa, for his immeasurable help in wading through medical jargon and for asking all the right questions, forcing me to address them honestly and accurately. Ricky Barker, a fellow writer and also author of an incredibly inspiring book, *A Reason to Believe*, who is always complimentary and encouraging—right-back-at-ya, Rick.

A big, humble "thanks" to Dr. Brian Forrest, MD, a healer and as improbable as it sounds these days, a great listener and literally my life support. He generously gave of his time to allow me to discuss my theories about autism, and gave helpful advice on how to research my theory on Agenesis of the Corpus Callosum.

And no one goes very far down life's highway without family or the friends who ran out for more paper, inkjet refills and diet Sprite. Thanks to J.B., my biggest fan. To Annie, who encourages me to "keep it real." To Michael, the tech support-computer whiz, who patiently helped with the recovery of my work and me.

Naturally, I can never forget my "home-townies," Brenda, Linda and Alice, thanks for the many hours when we sat on the porch and downed gallons of sweet tea. Y'all know I can never repay you, but if I could y'all would be filthy rich. Amen.

Made in the USA
Charleston, SC
18 October 2013